How to Keep Your Husband Alive!

Siegfried J. Kra
M.D., F.A.C.P
Assoc. Clinical Professor of Medicine
Yale School of Medicine

LF LEBHAR-FRIEDMAN BOOKS
NEW YORK · CHICAGO · LOS ANGELES · LONDON · PARIS · TOKYO

Copyright © 2002 Lebhar-Friedman Books

Lebhar-Friedman Books
425 Park Avenue
New York, NY 10022

Published by Lebhar-Friedman Books
Lebhar-Friedman Books is a company of
Lebhar-Friedman, Inc.

Printed in the United States of America

Library of Congress Cataloging-in-Publication Data
on file at the Library of Congress

ISBN: 0-86730-864-8

Visit our Web site at lfbooks.com

Contents

iii

CONTENTS

Acknowledgments

I wish to thank my agent Don Gasterwirth for his tireless encouragement and excellent job in editing this book. Also, my thanks go to all my patients who are not named in this book, and to my two daughters, Lisette and Arnice, and my significant other Lolita Pridgeon, for their intelligent and useful advice and critique.

Introduction

What can a woman do to extend the life of her spouse?

Would it not be wonderful if most men lived to a ripe old age along with their spouses? The sad fact of the matter is that most men don't.

It is unfair for women to be relegated to lives of loneliness after their mates die prematurely because of illness and neglect of their health.

Medical miracles are happening each day and new, exciting molecular biology investigations prepare us to live longer than ever before in history, often well into the next century. Most men neglect this new information, even at this moment, even though they know the number one killer of men is heart disease, followed by strokes and cancer.

Most of us do not like to be nagged or critiqued by our mates. We want to feel we are in control of our daily lives. At the same time it is a nice feeling to know that our mates want to see us healthy, and we like being comforted emotionally and, of course, physically.

The experience of thirty-eight years of medical practice, and attending to more than 100,000 patients has convinced me that a woman can help to extend her man's life by the simplest of ways—and not come across as sounding petulant or overbearing. It is an awesome responsibility that I am asking of the woman. First, she takes care of her children, runs a household, works at a job, is a full-time wife, and now I come along and suggest *another* task as critical as childcare.

For example, one of the most important early signs of something gone awry in our bodies is fatigue. At first it may be so insidious that only the spouse may notice that her husband looks tired. His eyes—the "mirror of the soul"—may not have that glow that she is used to seeing. Baseball player Yogi Berra put it simply—and I am paraphrasing—"If you don't look, you don't see." And the spouse usually can tell if she just looks. Or to quote the German poet Goethe, "What one knows one sees." Who knows her husband's constitution better than his wife? Besides losing the glow in her husband's eyes, are there a little more creases at the corner of the eyes? Are the eyelids drooping just a bit more? Look at the whites of his eyes; are they slightly red or, perhaps, somewhat pale? Some men's eye color actually may change before they become overtly ill—blue becomes pale, brown becomes less brown, or sometimes black. Then as more fatigue sets in the man, he might need to sleep just a little longer in the morning or he might start going to bed earlier and earlier. He may yawn, not out of displeasure or boredom, but because his body is exhausted or starved for air. He may sigh more than usual, not only because of contentment, or despair and frustration—but it also could be due to lack of oxygen.

Fatigue can be the earliest sign that a heart attack is about to take place. The arteries, called the coronary arteries, supply precious blood and oxygen to the heart, and are slowly being dammed up by nefarious cholesterol plaques and other notorious substances. Ever so slowly, the blood is impeded in its flow. The body cries out for oxygen. The message is sent to the brain: Not enough blood is coming to the heart. The heart cannot tolerate this insult and reduces the amount of blood that it delivers to the brain and vital organs. Fatigue sets in and increases relentlessly until suddenly it is replaced by breathing difficulties. An ominous chest pain springs up from out of nowhere as the blockage suddenly strikes like lightning. Again the spouse has the opportunity to save her husband's life. How? Read on.

Fatigue can also be the harbinger of cancer, infections, metabolic problems, and depression.

So often in my practice I hear (after a catastrophic event), "Actually, he has been looking and acting tired for months. I thought it was because he had to work longer hours and was traveling a lot more." I am referring to prolonged fatigue that may become worse as each day passes.

Exhaustion likewise belongs in the same group of symptoms that signals possible impending disaster. The lawn was left half-mowed or there is unfinished work at the office: There's no longer a careful line-up of shoes and socks according to the day of the week, etc. These may be signs of his being too tired to do the usual tasks.

What should the spouse NOT do after she has noticed these changes?

Spouse: "Are you feeling all right?"
Man: "Why? What's wrong? What did I do now?"
Spouse: "Nothing, you just don't seem right. Your closet is a mess, your papers are all over the house. You look sick to me."

Man: "There is nothing wrong with me so stop bugging me—I will clean the mess."

As a result of this type of conversation, there will be a delay before the man sees a doctor who would discover early that his coronary arteries slowly closing off.

What SHOULD the spouse do and say?

Spouse: "Dear, you know I love you very much, and who knows you better than me, right? Well, it is not like you to not finish up what you start. You are a hard worker, a quality which I admire in you."

Man: "What do you mean, 'not finishing'? Well I just didn't feel like doing the usual today. Big deal!"

Spouse: "No big deal, dear. I just have a feeling that perhaps it is time to call for your checkup. You know, your yearly."

Man: "I do feel just a bit out of sorts—I will go and see Dr. G. I will make the appointment as soon as I get a chance."

Spouse: "Dear, I wanted to save you the trouble—I know how busy you are—so I made the appointment for you. You have two dates to choose from next week."

Now this does not end here, because the wife knows—as I will discuss later—that an EKG has limited value. She can ask the doctor if a chest X-ray and stress test would be appropriate, in the event the busy HMO doctor does not recommend it. Having him see the doctor early could save her spouse's life.

Other early signs of illness are:

- Color of the face: pale, blue lips. Red face, yellow tinge
- Bad breath
- Hair loss
- Sudden onset of shortness of breath
- Indigestion or heartburn
- Loss of appetite for specific foods
- Weight gain or weight loss
- Diarrhea, constipation, or blood in stool
- Increased frequency of urination (i.e., up at night more than usual)
- Loss of libido or impotence
- Mood swings, anger, or depression
- Dependency, and fear of being alone
- Increased or decreased use of alcohol

I wish to make the spouse a surrogate for the intelligent, observing doctor who sometimes may be so "HMOized" that he fails in his job to detect a disease early.

What else can the spouse do to save the life of her husband?

A sensible, proper diet—one that is eatable and *not* a punishment for being alive—can be a lifesaver. I have a simple, wonderful diet called the Kra Diet that reduces all the bad things that kill when consumed in excess—fat, cholesterol, and sugar. It's a diet that anyone can prepare, and it's not time-consuming. I have been using this diet in my practice for thirty years and it works. There are no gimmicks in this diet, no supplements that I sell from my closet, and no questionable natural additives.

Besides infection, smoking is probably the number one killer in the world. The spouse can save her smoking man's life if she becomes involved in the stop-smoking program discussed later in this book.

There is a desperate need to put into perspective the real truths and myths about all the magical supplements advocated by the special interest groups and the companies that promote them.

What should you put on the breakfast table for the man in your life—one, ten, fifteen pills or more, bought without prescription? Pills for the urine, pills for the penis, pills to prevent cancer, pills to prevent arteriosclerosis, pills for depression, pills for memory loss? I ask my male patients, "Do you take any vitamins? If so, which ones?" Answer: "Doc, I don't know which vitamins they are; whatever my wife puts on the table I take. I leave it all to her." Be cautious! Some supplements are dangerous and you should be aware of the consequences of all those bottles you leave in front of your husband at breakfast. I will give you guidelines to what is considered to be useful, based on real scientific studies and not chimerical speculations.

A good sex life is essential for healthy males and females. I will discuss this delicate subject, incorporating all that I have heard and learned in confidence during thirty-eight years of medical practice and innumerable conferences with other physicians and professionals.

Finally, I have written nine books over the last two decades—and none has had the life-saving potential as the one I set before you now.

—Siegfried J. Kra, M.D., F.A.C.P.

Grow old along with me,
The best is yet to be.
The last of life,
for which the first was made.

"Rabbi Ben Ezra"
by Robert Browning

Chapter One

What the Spouse Should Know About Herbs & Herbal Medicine

MANY PRODUCTS bought over-the-counter and in health stores can cause a catastrophe when mixed with prescribed medications.

Some common foods, such as a bowl of oatmeal or bran cereal, and St. John's wort taken along with a heart drug called digoxin (Lanoxin) could lead to inadequate dosage. Digoxin is used for heart failure and irregular heart beats.

Inadequate dosage as well as too much of a drug can make a medical condition worse than what it would be if you did not take the medications.

We recently discovered that grapefruit juice taken with cholesterol-lowering drugs can cause high levels of these drugs. Antibiotics such as Cipro or tetracycline taken with calcium-fortified orange juice may decrease the absorption of these medications and delay the cure of the infections. Thyroid hormones that have been prescribed for an under-active thyroid should not be taken at the same time with minerals such as calcium or iron, as they interfere with the absorption of the replacement hormone. The doctor might then keep increasing the dosage of the medications because the level, when measured by the laboratory, was not achieved.

Bill was diagnosed with an underactive thyroid and his doctor gave him thyroid replacement. The doctor had to keep increasing the dosage of the thyroid medications as the thyroid remained underactive and the doctor feared either he was not taking the medication or the diagnosis was not correct. The patient's spouse insisted that she gave the medication to her husband every morning at breakfast. She finally added, "He takes all his medications along with a calcium pill and iron; I thought he could use calcium as he gets older."

Once Bill stopped taking calcium pills his thyroid medications started to work.

Another culprit that can affect the absorption of medications is coffee; it reduces the absorption of the drug cimetidine and the antibiotic Cipro if taken at the same time.

Coumadin, a medication essential to prevent blood clots, is also a dangerous drug as it can cause bleeding in the brain and anywhere in the body if the dosage is too high, or if combined with aspirin, for example. I will discuss these issues in greater detail in forthcoming chapters. Suffice it to say that if you take Coumadin and eat a spinach omelet, the spinach can block the action of the Coumadin, and medications such as Prilosec (for reflux) can cause too much Coumadin in the blood and bleeding can result. Over-the-counter drugs that can interfere with Coumadin are Vitamin K, Vitamin D, Vitamin E, Bromelain, dan shen (a Chinese herb), garlic, and gingko biloba. Ginger, garlic, and feverfew (an herb used for migraine) can also be the culprit. Recently I was invited to dine with a very wealthy man who was on Coumadin and the conversation, as always, turned to medicine. His doctor, a renowned cardiologist, had trouble regulating his Coumadin dosage. "Are you taking any herbs?" I asked my host. He hesitated and said, "Isn't everybody?" It turned out that he was taking excess garlic and ginger but his doctor never asked if he was taking any over-the-counter substances. As soon as he stopped taking the garlic and ginger he stopped having small amounts of bleeding and his INR was controlled. There are dozens upon dozens of prescribed medications that can interfere with Coumadin. Make sure you ask your physician what they are.

ACETAMINOPHEN

Acetaminophen (or Tylenol, as it is most marketed) is one of the most common over-the-counter medications used in America. It is found in hundreds of compounds purported to remedy colds, fever, headaches, and arthritic pains. Many people take it every day.

Does the following story resonate to you? The millennium party was a great success. Actually it was a two-day celebration with martinis, champagne, wines, and after-dinner drinks. The dinner might well be remembered for years to come. Starting with three martinis and white wine with oysters, the best Bordeaux with the roast, and then the best Napoleon brandy with the Cuban cigars. The party was, needless to say, a little intoxicating. The truth of the matter, to be told, was that each weekend Jack had martinis and wine—but since this was a special time, he had more than his usual. After all, it was a celebration for a new millennium, and business was "*comme il faut*", as the French would say. The morning after, Jack and his wife—who were a happy couple with grown children and great success in the stock market—were having their usual breakfast: bran enriched with folic acid and covered with soy milk, a tall glass of fresh orange juice, and bran bread with honey. "Jack," his wife, Jill, spoke lovingly, "You look really tired and you are holding your head."

"Yes," Jack muttered, "my head is killing me."

On the table was a basket packed with ten different bottles of herbs. "Take a couple of these acetaminophen compounds; they will help." Jack took two and two more in a few hours and again two more after that. Three days later Jill noticed Jack's eyes were yellow and his urine was brown. Jill suspected Jack had acute hepatitis and the liver expert Jack finally visited agreed with the diagnosis. Unfortunately Jill, nor Jack, did not know that the acetaminophen compounds and alcohol caused the hepatitis. It is called the alcohol-acetaminophen syndrome. The experts tell us that *it does not* take many acetaminophens to cause hepatitis in susceptible people.

Beware! Alcohol and the headache pill taken together can be dangerous to your health. It does not belong on the breakfast table if you are a chronic, moderate, or heavy alcohol drinker. Moderate drinker means one or two drinks per day. The liver can be so destroyed that only a liver transplant can save the life.

VITAMIN E, VITAMIN C, & BETA CAROTENE

At a recent conference I asked my fellow doctors how many were taking Vitamin E, Vitamin C and beta carotene daily to prevent heart disease and strokes? Everyone in the audience raised their hands.

That same week there were reports on how beneficial Vitamin E is for the prevention of heart disease and stroke. However, a report in the *Annals of Internal Medicine*, 1999, involving 43,738 male health professionals during a two-year study did not show a decrease of strokes reported.

Still another recent report from the *New England Journal of Medicine* showed that Vitamin E did not reduce the risk of heart attack or stroke, and was not recommended as a preventative. I no longer recommend Vitamin E to my patients for this purpose.

ASPIRIN

Big Stanley, as I call him, had a slow heartbeat and he had a tendency toward low blood pressure. Surely, Big Stanley who is 75 would some day need a pacemaker to keep his heart rate normal. One afternoon, Big Stanley came to my clinic because he had almost collapsed while gardening.

We found his heart rate was 45 and his blood pressure was down to 100/70. I decided to place a Holter monitor on his chest to monitor his heart for 24 hours to see if his heart rate dropped to below 45 and caused the symptoms he described to me.

As he was leaving my office I asked if he was taking aspirin. "Of course I am. I take a baby aspirin three times a week to prevent a heart attack," he said. Just to be sure, I performed a rectal examination on Big Stanley and found his stools were black as charcoal, and the test was positive for blood. Big Stanley was bleeding internally and needed three pints of blood—it was not his heart that caused him to feel faint and nearly collapse, but internal bleeding caused by aspirin. He told the staff at Yale New Haven Hospital that he self-prescribed aspirin after hearing the Bayer aspirin commercial on television!

Aspirin has been used as a pain reliever for 2,500 years. It is an herb originally derived from willow bark. Pliny the Elder used it for back pain, and American Indians made tea from the bark to relieve fever. In 1892, chemist Felix Hoffman refined pure aspirin for his father-in-law to relieve his pain from arthritis. Hoffman then sold the refined product to Bayer Company of Germany.

The British chemist, noble laureate Sir John Vane discovered how aspirin works. It stops the production of an enzyme called COX, which in turn stops the production of prostaglandins that contribute to pain, swelling, and fever. Thromboxane, another prostaglandin, is responsible for platelets sticking together and causing blood clots. Aspirin inhibits thromboxane production with the result that platelets don't stick together in a gluey mess. It takes ten days for the effects of aspirin to wear off.

Aspirin is recommended for men who have risk factors like smoking, high cholesterol, a strong family history of heart attacks, and those who had a previous heart attack.

It is a potentially dangerous drug for the stomach and intestines because it can cause serious bleeding. Bleeding from the gastrointestinal tract carries a very high mortality rate, up to 40 percent in an elderly person.

I favor using a low dosage of aspirin, 80 mg every other day for men at risk of a heart attack or stroke.

If your spouse takes aspirin every other day, make sure he reports black stools or bleeding from the rectum, and seeks immediate attention.

If your spouse is having a heart attack let him chew on an aspirin, preferably not coated aspirin, as it works faster on the way to the hospital. Aspirin lowers the death rate by 25 percent and the risk of a second heart attack by 50 percent.

CALCIUM

It is not uncommon for older women to take calcium tablets if they have lactose intolerance or are postmenopausal and want to preserve their bones.

Avery, who subscribes to every magazine that features articles on how to live longer and better, read that men suffer from osteoporosis, like women, and need calcium. Avery shares calcium pills along with Vitamin E, Vitamin C, and a dozen other "magical" pills with his wife, Hillary. It takes them as long to swallow the pills as to eat their breakfast. I had the feeling he would have liked to share her estrogen pills as well.

"It has become like a religious crusade," says Walter Willingness, professor and chairman of the Department of Nutrition at Harvard School of Public Health. "The need to increase calcium intake simply is not based on sound data."

Now Avery is also one of these guys who buys foods fortified with calcium such as Tropicana orange juice, Viactic calcium chocolates, Shedd's Spread margarine with calcium added, Breyers calcium-enriched ice-cream, and antacids like Tums and Mylanta for the heartburn he gets from Viactic chocolate!

Avery started to act strangely, his wife Hillary told me. He had become depressed because in another few months he was scheduled to get the "golden handshake" from his Washington based PR firm. He was always complaining of stomach cramps, numbness of his feet and hands, he had become constipated, he was urinating a lot, and he was always thirsty.

At three o'clock in the morning one day my telephone rang. It was Hillary, telling me Avery had severe pain in his stomach. In the emergency room we discovered Avery had suffered a severe attack of kidney stones. The stones were calcium stones and his calcium level was 18 (normal is below five).

After his calcium stone attack was over, we cautioned Hillary and Avery to stay away from calcium pills and calcium supplements, and the 234 food and beverages enriched with calcium that the industry has introduced since 1995.

Men are cautioned on taking excess calcium pills, as there is some relationship between prostate cancer, bone fractures, and high calcium intake. Excess calcium causes kidney stones and kidney failure, depression, headaches, and chronic irritability.

Once Avery's calcium level returned to normal he became the delightful, charming man he was before, and was looking forward to his early retirement.

FOLIC ACID

This is a vitamin that is useful to take if you have elevated levels of homocysteine in the blood. Men and women who have elevated levels of homocysteine in the blood have a marked increase in arteriosclerosis of the heart and the arteries of the brain and legs. Folic acid and Vitamin B6 and Vitamin B1 help to decrease the homocytseine level to normal. The dosage is probably around 500 mcg per day to bring down the homocysteine level.

I will discuss Homocysteine Theory in greater detail further on in the text on heart disease.

VITAMIN C

Without Vitamin C a terrible deadly disease called scurvy sets in. It was the dreaded disease among sailors until 1639 when John Woodall, a British physician, recommended drinking lemon juice to avoid scurvy. It took another hundred years for Captain James Cook to issue lime juice to the sailors to avoid scurvy. Hence the slang term "Limey" for someone from Britain. Progress was slow in medicine and several hundred years had to pass before the American-Hungarian chemist Stent Gyŏrgi stated that Vitamin C could help prevent scurvy.

Then there was the famous two-time Nobel Prize winner, Linus Pauling, who advocated thousands of mg of Vitamin C for a long, good life. He died at the age of 92 from leukemia.

Supplements of Vitamin C are pretty much the norm these days as nutritionists and chemists tell us that so much of the vitamin is destroyed by cooking and refining our food. Furthermore, as we do not eat enough fresh fruits, our intake of Vitamin C is inadequate.

Many years ago, in a hospital intensive care unit, I saw my first case of scurvy. A patient was hospitalized for almost a month in a coma. His mouth was filled with blood one morning and his gums were swollen. He was receiving intravenous fluids and protein mixtures. When I checked the formula of the mixture I realized it did not contain Vitamin C. Once he received the vitamin, the bleeding from his mouth ceased, and he recovered from his stroke.

Now here comes the clincher! At the annual conference of cardiovascular disease epidemiology and prevention, sponsored by the American Heart Association, Dr. James Dwyer, Ph.D., reported that supplements of Vitamin C might accelerate arteriosclerosis in the carotid artery!

Similar findings that rocked the preventive cardiology world were reported by a Finnish group that found that beta-carotene vitamin supplements resulted in an increase in mortality rather than a decrease.

You can't beat fresh fruits and fresh squeezed oranges on the breakfast table to get your Vitamin C—then there is no need to take Vitamin C supplements.

HERBAL MEDICINE

On July 6, 1999, it was reported in *The New York Times*, "Doctors emphasize that much study needs to be done to establish whether there is a real risk for patients taking herbal remedies."

Herbal products are not regulated by the federal government, as are prescription drugs. The American public spends $5 billion annually on herbal products.

Herbal remedies have been with us at least 5,000 years, dating back to the earliest days of Ayurvedic and Chinese medicine. There must be something to these preparations if they existed for so long without the serious toxic effects we hear about now.

Recently, Dr. John B. Neeld, Jr., president of the American Society of Anesthesiologists, issued a warning to consumers using herbs that some may have serious interactions with the drugs used to anesthetize patients during surgery. St. John's wort, gingko, feverfew, and ephedra were shown to cause a serious drop in blood pressure and bleeding during anesthesia.

Herbal products once harvested fresh can be eaten whole or mixed in food. Herbs are dried, sold in bulk, prepared in tea, infusions, or tinctures and sold as capsules. There are no controls on how much active ingredients exist in these capsules.

I have known patients to take 20 to 30 herbal medications each morning at breakfast. Yet some of these same patients complain bitterly about the cost of prescribed medications for their heart and blood pressure. I have stood and watched consumers at health food stores spend $100 to $200 at a clip for dozens of herbal products. Madison Avenue is on a rush to advertise by mail, video, radio, and TV. Media offer products to help your sex life or to prevent aging or cancer. In spite of all these good intentions, cancer is on the increase; heart attacks, strokes, AIDS, suicides, and drug addictions are epidemic. Obesity is also on the rise. I happen to know smokers who take Vitamin E to allegedly prevent the cancer and heart disease often associated with smoking. A recent study in the prestigious *New England Journal of Medicine* questioned whether Vitamin E has an effect on preventing heart attacks or other vascular complications. In another study from Finland, participants taking Vitamin E actually had a higher incidence of lung cancer.

We have blaring examples of great leaders, men and women of immense wealth, falling prey to charlatans who dish out magical cures and treatments to prolong life. President Kennedy used to get novacaine injections in New York from Doctor Feelgood who after many years finally lost his license to practice. Other illustrious persons did the same—Pope Pious V, Winston Churchill, and Konrad Adenauer all sought out alternative medicine.

GINGKO BILOBA

Gingko is the world's oldest tree; it grows in China and has been used in Chinese medicine for 4,000 years to improve breathing and brain function. The remaining species of the family Gingkoacea is believed to be 200 million years old. It was brought to the United States in 1784.

Research on gingko has been conducted since 1950 to study its potential to enhance mental performance and ameliorate symptoms of cerebral vascular insufficiency, known today as TIA—dizzy spells, numbness of arms, legs, face, weak spells, and memory loss resulting from inadequate blood flow to the brain.

Some recent studies demonstrate gingko's effectiveness in improving geriatric depression. In uncomplicated early dementia, gingko improved vigilance, sociability, mood behavior, and cognitive function.

For peripheral vascular insufficiency—poor arterial blood flow to the legs which causes cramps and pain on walking—patients using 160 mg/day of gingko biloba had a marked improvement, and were judged to have longer walking distances without pain. European studies found that this herb, given over prolonged periods of time, increases the flow of blood in the leg arteries.

Studies are in progress in Boston to determine if this herb is just another placebo, or if it is truly a beneficial substance to allay the diseases of older men and women: depression, dementia, stroke, and vascular illness.

The reader must be warned, however, that gingko is a drug that can cause severe deadly hemorrhages to the brain if taken with the anticoagulant Coumadin or warfarin. It also causes headaches and dizziness in some sensitive persons.

ST. JOHN'S WORT
(Hypericum perfoatum)

This pretty blue flowering plant is grown all over the world. It had magic powers in medieval Europe, or so claimed herbalists. It could soften the cold hearts of shrewish maidens and bring new life to shriveled old men. This flower decorated the churches and halls of castles for the feast of St. John the Baptist. "Wort" is the Old English word for plant.

Today in Europe, it is prescribed seven times more often than fluoxetine (the current popular antidepressant medication) for mild to moderate depression. The use of St. John's wort (SJW) in the United States has increased from $20 million to $200 million between 1995 and 1997.

In twenty-three random trials, which involved 1,757 subjects with depression, SJW was significantly better than a placebo.

How does this magical herb work? This herb affects three mechanisms responsible for depression as used by conventional antidepressant medications. They inhibit reuptake of seratonin, norephenepherine, and dopamine. Depression can occur if levels of all three compounds are low in the body. Also, it reduces the number of seratonin receptors, thus more seratonin becomes available. The active ingredient of St. John's wort is hypericin (along with many other substances that inhibit the uptake of various neurotransmitters involved in depression).

So far, drug interactions have not been reported and the only side effect, described in 6 percent of patients, is some gastrointestinal upset. Caution has been advised, though, in being exposed to ultraviolet therapy while taking SJW. The use of St. John's wort and other antidepressant medications should be closely monitored since hyperforin is the main active ingredient in all antidepressant medications.

A word of caution to the spouse who sees her or his mate become depressed. Depression is a potentially serious illness, too often fatal, and should not be managed alone with an herb, but requires expert diagnosis and treatment outlined by a qualified therapist and/or a physician.

ECHINACEA
(E. Angustifolia, E. Pallida, E. Purpurea, Purple Coneflower)

Native Americans have used the plant for centuries.

The active ingredients consist of flavenoids, polysaccharides, essential oils, alkyl amides, and caffeic acids. The root is being used to enhance the immune system. Subjects with colds were given the root and the recovery time was reduced by four days. There were no side effects or drug interactions with this root when it was given in the dosage of 3 ml of tincture, three times per day, diluted.

Although there are three-hundred controlled studies, the size of each study involved a relatively small number of patients, and the data is difficult to interpret. I don't prescribe it.

GARLIC
(Allium sativum)

Garlic was described 5,000 years ago in the Egyptian medical papyrus. Louis Pasteur, who discovered the first treatment for syphilis, noted the garlic antibiotic activity.

Garlic, grown originally in central Asia, is a member of the lily family named Allin, a sulfur component known to be chiefly responsible for its medicinal effect.

Garlic is alleged to lower cholesterol, treat high blood pressure, help leg circulation, and cure infections. The studies are conflicting and controversial, but it is definitely an antiplatlet compound and should be avoided before surgery as it can cause too much bleeding. And if you are taking Coumadin, beware—it can cause bleeding.

Does it belong on the breakfast table? It will depend on which study you read and believe. I, for one, prefer it on the dinner table with my salad, or with veal scallopini.

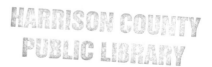

ALOE VERA
(A. vulgari and A. barbadensis)

This plant dates back to 170 B.C. in Mesopotamia—often an area of conflict, where bitter wars were fought and men suffered horrible injuries from dirty, blunt instruments. The injuries would, of course, become infected, oozing pus and emitting a putrid odor. Along came one of the healers with his own secret plant root. It was boiled in water with dried leaves. The concoction was then placed on the wounds of the injured warrior. The wound began to heal with the aloe vera. It was also used as a last resort cathartic for chronic constipation.

Its healing power comes from the anthraquinones, saccharides, prostaglandin, and fatty acids.

It is also used for the unfortunate soul who gets too much sun. Some physicians have used the gel for the treatment of peptic ulcer and psoriasis.

CHAMOMILE
(Matricaria recutia)

This herb grows wild in all temperate climates and its flower heads have been used medicinally ever since the first century A.D.

When I was a child my mother used to take the chamomilian leaves and make a tea that she used for gastrointestinal distress and when her nerves got the best of her. It worked. There are no contradictions or side effects known from this herb. It is safe to take to relieve anxiety.

PEPPERMINT
(Mentha piperita)

Everyone knows about peppermint in all its forms as a candy or as an oil for steam inhaling: It's also often used for bloating and colic.

It was discovered by the Egyptians; it was found in their pyramids, dating back to 1000 B.C. Peppermint products relax the lower esophageal sphincter.

But don't put this on the breakfast table if your spouse or significant other has trouble with their gall bladder or if they have liver damage or a common illness known as GERD (or gastrointestinal reflux disease). The symptoms of GERD are heartburn and indigestion, so if you give them peppermint drops it will make the indigestion worse. And if there is gall bladder disease, it can cause more obstruction of the flow of bile.

ALTERNATIVE SUPPLEMENTARY PILLS AND FOOD are just beginning to be taken seriously by federal investigators. Once genuine studies have been completed—*preferably studies not sponsored by the food and vitamin industry*—then we all can be reassured of their real value in our daily living.

Do they prevent disease? Do they prolong our lives? Are they really safe? These are the questions I ask in my own life before I decide to take supplements. Once I wrote that the use of tryptophane for sleep, as the naturopaths and others advocated it, is worth a try—later it turned out to cause blood diseases, and tryptophane was soon taken off the market!

Chapter Two

What IS the Difference Between Men and Women?

IT IS THEIR HORMONES. Men have predominantly testosterone and women have mostly estrogen. Sometimes they both have equal proportions of both and then things really get confusing. Men produce 15 to 20 times more testosterone than women and this chemical determines the physique, mood, and behavior of men. Testosterone was isolated in 1935, and synthesized by Adolph Butenandt in Germany in 1936.

In the male, the major manufacture of testosterone takes place in the testes. These organs hang outside of the body because the temperature within the body is too hot for the sperm, which they produce, to survive.

In 1771, John Hunter, the renowned scientist, gave thought to what makes a male a male. He transplanted the testes of a cock into hens and watched the masculine effects. The hens acted like roosters. This was the same doctor who infected himself with syphilis from a diseased patient to prove how the disease is transmitted. In 1889, Brown-Sequard, the renowned French physiologist, injected himself with testicular extract to gain vigor and capacity for work. We then learned the extract contained male hormones. Since these first experiments were performed, hundreds of thousands of other experiments followed, demonstrating conclusively that male hormones, such as testosterone and androgen, are responsible for the male characteristics.

At birth, the peanut-size testes secrete small amounts of male hormones until puberty, and then the boy becomes a man in the chemical sense. The penis and scrotum grow, pubic hair surfaces, and there is a rapid increase in height and development of the musco-skeletal system. The skin becomes thicker and oily, surface fat is lost, veins become prominent, underarm hair grows, as well as hair on the chest and pelvis. Early on, puberty erections are frequent, as is masturbation. Growth of a beard occurs much later.

Testosterone is the principal male hormone. Daily, 7 mg of it is produced by a man's outdoor pharmaceutical plant located in the hanging testes of the scrotum. The other male hormones, called androgens—about 10 percent of which are made internally—are produced by the adrenal gland. Men make estrogen from sources outside of the testes.

Women produce male hormones in the ovary, including 0.5 mg of testosterone daily. The ovary is also the site for the formation of estrogen and progesterone. The placenta and the adrenal glands also make estrogen, and so do other tissues and organs, such as the liver, muscle, and hair follicles.

Estrogen is remarkably similar in chemical structure to testosterone. Both chemical structures are rings differing by a small molecule called an OH, which is missing on the male ring. At puberty, estrogen is responsible for growth, and the development of the vagina, uterus, fallopian tubes, and breasts. Growth of auxiliary and public hair; pigmentation of the skin, nipples, and aureole; and responsibility for the menstrual cycle are the results of estrogen secretions. Breast development is first seen in the beginning of puberty, followed by the appearance of pubic hair. This is followed, usually two years later, by the menarche (the first menstrual period), usually between the ages of 8 and 14. Puberty in the male usually occurs between the age of 12 and 14. The lean body mass and body fat are about equal in males and females during pre-puberty, but by puberty women have twice as much body fat and less lean skeletal and muscle mass than men.

Prior to puberty, both sexes have a tendency to be similar. "Gender-neutral" styling emerged around age 5 and 6. The toy marketers for decades avoided boy-girl stereotypes, which, of course, has now changed. The notion once rang through the toy world that "Boys and girls are the same." Some parents today are upset with the new notion of a boys' world and girls' world. An article in the *Wall Street Journal*, published on February 14, 2000, discusses the brand-new strategy of toy manufactures to make toys gender-orientated, and to acknowledge male-female differences. Manufacturers have stayed with the notion that "boys will be boys and girls will be both." You can sell a boy's product to a girl, but not the reverse. Boys become hostile if girls invade their space. Fox's new digital cable channels feature patterns for boys and girls. You don't need a therapist to tell the difference between men and women, just take notice of the interest in the video stores. Men gravitate towards *Gladiator*, *Star Wars*, or any James Bond films—and women tend to go for *Sophie's Choice*, *Little Women*, or *Love Story*.

Men remain aggressive and combative from childhood to manhood. Separation of the genders continues almost in epidemic fashion. More and more TV shows are devoted solely to women; men have the History Channel or sports. War movies and cowboy films are viewed mainly by males. On one hand, society stresses well-deserved equality of women and men in all aspects of our world such as women in combat and sports, and, at the same time, advertises the marvelous differences between the genders.

We have now moved to an open society with the advertising of products for feminine hygiene and jock itch treatment for men. And now these commercials can be broadcast in an open forum to everyone, even children. The six o'clock news can advertise treatments for men who fail to get an erection— what the sponsors charmingly call "erectile dysfunction." Even retired senators tell us of their sexual inabilities. For now at least, I have not seen any advertisements on TV for women's sexual problems, such as the inability to achieve an orgasm or products for painful intercourse or lack of sexual desire.

Although women have long been labeled as the weaker sex, perhaps because estrogen makes their skin softer and more sensitive, this, too, is a wrongful assumption. Ask any experienced nurse who works in the hospital regarding the pain tolerance of men as compared to women. Men become much more frightened and more childlike when it comes to pain. All the machismo of men, on the surface, swiftly dissipates like a tired fog. Women learn to endure pain through their own childbirth experience. A lot of men are sensitive and cry at movies, their daughters' weddings, or when they see their grandchild for the first time. In many other cultures, as in France, Spain, or Italy, men show their emotions in public; heterosexual males can be seen on the streets or in the cafe kissing and hugging each other whenever they meet or part. In the United States, one rarely sees two American-born males openly be affectionate to each other. The first time I was hugged and kissed by a Russian colleague, in a ward of Yale

New Haven Hospital after not seeing him for ten years, I was so embarrassed that I wanted to climb under a stretcher. We always see women kissing each other in public and don't give it a second thought.

Many old black-and-white movies made the man appear strong, brave, and wise, and the woman quiet and submissive. As the bullet or arrow is removed from the cowboy's chest, he is told to bite the bullet placed between his teeth to ward off the screams and endure the excruciating pain that will follow. Compare this picture to a James Bond movie where the nefarious killer is a powerful woman who can toss James Bond fifty feet, or to Catwoman attacking Batman. Women, indeed, can be stronger than men can. In fact, many are.

When I was an undergraduate at CCNY, I had a chemistry professor who was the most despotic, cruel, and miserable human being I ever met. He taught our advanced physical chemistry class and during our final examination before Christmas, he sat and watched us struggle as he puffed on his cigarette, blowing smoke in our faces. "Bring any book you wish, or a genius to help you with these finals." The questions were almost impossible to answer. I had two open books on my desk; others brought more. The following day, before Christmas Eve, we came to the laboratories, terrified, to learn of the test results. On each lab table there was a bottle of scotch, glasses, cookies, and cigars. He marched into the laboratory with the usual frown on his face, as we all stood astounded. He spoke in his habitual quiet creepy tone, "Merry Christmas. I know you are all cut from the same cloth." And he walked out of the laboratory saying no more. We all passed our exams with good grades and were admitted to medical school. This nefarious-acting macho man, whom we feared, turned out to be a very sensitive human being.

What he meant in saying "from the same cloth," was that we students from poor families came to CCNY on scholarship.

Many men, who pretend to be brave and nonchalant when faced with such warnings of imminent illness, no matter how bad things are, insist on saying, "I am fine." These three words have caused more disabilities and deaths than the reader will ever imagine. The man now sets up an entire denial system for several reasons. It may be that he does not want anyone to know that he is ill and then fears he will lose his role as master of his ship, so to speak. Businessmen and professionals are legion to hide their symptoms and illness. In plain truth, they lie (and lie to themselves and the doctor).

I have for many years now performed preflight pilot examinations, which should include a complete physical examination and heart test. One pilot I examined was a former naval test pilot hired by a corporation to fly their executives. He denied smoking cigarettes but the odor of tobacco on his body was distinctive, and the tips of his fingers were brown from tobacco stains. He also denied drinking, and alcohol was on his breath.

"You don't drink, yet I detect alcohol on your breath." He answered, "Doc, I use an alcohol-based mouthwash, that is what you smell."

"But I also detect cigar smoke on your body," I challenged him.

"Listen, Doc, my whole house smells like a smoke factory, my wife is a chain smoker and won't stop."

I examined the pilot who, except for some rare wheezes in his chest, appeared normal. "You will have a stress test and chest X-ray and blood work next," I told him. "Doc, I have to fly my boss to L.A. in one hour; schedule me for next week. I will do the stress test next time, but I will get the chest X-ray now." As he left my office, after his chest X-ray was taken in our X-ray department, he looked a little pale but was gone before I could schedule him for the stress test. His wife called me shortly later. "Did you see my husband, Mitch, the pilot? Did he tell you he has had chest pain and coughing for two weeks? I am sure he didn't. I wanted to come with him because I knew he would lie to you."

I hurried to the X-ray department and saw that his chest X-ray showed a large tumor and his blood test showed anemia. His EKG was normal. By now he was flying toward Los Angeles with his boss and three other executives. I called the company and the FAA, who in turn demanded Mitch land his plane at the nearest airport, which was at Oxford airfield in Connecticut. After he landed his plane, an ambulance was waiting for him; it took him to Yale New Haven Hospital.

Mitch died three hours later in spite of our efforts. If he or his wife had acted upon his chest pains, his life could have been saved. Luckily, we were able to bring him down just in time, because the other three people would have died with him. Mitch was afraid to tell anyone of his cough and chest pain because he did not want to lose his job and be grounded.

"I told him he should see a doctor," the wife told us later, "but he kept saying 'Stop nagging me, I am fine.'"

This unfortunate man knew very well what was happening to him, but he thought he could overcome it because his job was his life, and he was afraid to lose his job.

Tall, strong, silent types, as portrayed on the screen in *The Virginian* or *Shane*, were our heroes. We were brought up on these wonderful movies, with heroes who did not communicate with each other except with grunts and a blazing gun. In reality, most men tend to be lonely souls, and they share screams of approval or disappointment at football and basket-ball games—of course there are shouts of anger at their children and wives, but they don't talk to each other about their inner pains and frustrations. They might share some of their thoughts with their accountants, stockbrokers, or maybe a lawyer or two, and the few fortunate ones who can talk with their wives, and eventually with their psychiatrists.

Men do not listen—either to their wives or other men. "Hey, how are you?" one man asks another. Before he can answer the man who asked the question is already on another subject.

Suppose the man would answer, "I feel miserable; I am tired and I want to talk to you; I have some serious problems."

"Well, sure, why not call me tonight and we can talk."

"No, I must talk to you now."

This conversation rarely happens. Perhaps with email there will be talking and listening.

There is another major difference between the genders: Many women have friends who listen, and discuss intimate things with each other. They listen to each other but sometimes have a difficult time listening to a man, especially the man who begins each morning with the same complaint: "My back is killing me" or "All my joints hurt." Women have a marvelous support system that exists for each other. Women have less of a problem being intimate with each other. They have their own language that men can't understand. For men, perhaps their barber or bartender are the good listeners, and of course there are lucky men who have understanding and attentive wives or significant others.

Men claim to have all the answers—the diagnosis and the treatment. Many men who are not professionals but read *The*

Wall Street Journal or *The New York Times* and other sources of medical information act like they have the wisdom of Solomon. Thus, they will self-diagnose and treat, often using herbal or other inadequate cures. Women have less of a tendency to self-diagnose, but they, too, will see their gynecologist and then use herbal remedies, or even see a naturopath who will prescribe homeopathic remedies.

Every doctor's office will see twice as many women as it does men. As a rule, women pay much more attention to their discomforts and symptoms, and don't wait until the midnight hour to seek help.

Doctor C. was on vacation in the mountains; a superb cardiologist in our Yale community, he strolled through the forest in the Catskills. He started to have heartburn, swallowed antacid pills and then felt some relief. He reasoned that the heartburn came from the pizza he ate the night before. The following day he had a similar episode, ignored it and again self-diagnosed the discomfort as acid indigestion. A few days later he decided to visit the local emergency room because his heartburn became much worse. His wife knew of his heartburn but she too brushed it aside as indigestion. What makes this story so very painful is that his wife, too, was a physician.

The emergency room doctor diagnosed a massive heart attack and Dr. C. succumbed that same day. Could the wife have saved his life if she insisted he seek quicker medical attention? So often in my practice the spouse laments, "If only I insisted that he see a doctor, but he wouldn't listen to me."

I asked several senior wives, what was their secret in dealing with their stubborn macho men. They all answered the same thing: "Let him think he is the macho man. See to it that his clothes are clean, he has food on the table, and give him lots of sex if he wants it—and he does what I want him to and I let him feel he is the boss."

Another patient told me, "He is a stubborn, thick-headed man; he knew I was right. We went skiing in Aspen and he became lightheaded (as you would expect at that high altitude) when we were staying at the Jerome in Aspen, and still two days later he was dizzy and short of breath. I did not like the way he looked and simply packed all our bags and drove him to the local hospital. He was yelling and screaming how dare I force him to do this. In the hospital the chest X-ray revealed his lung to be collapsed. They kept him in for several days. After the doctor placed a chest tube, the chest expanded again and home we went. End of story. Now he listens to me and that is why I brought him in for a checkup."

In summary, men tend to be selfish, testosterone-driven, stubborn, controlling, angry, poor listeners, aggressive, sometimes potentially brutal—quite opposite to most women. Men tend to be mechanically inclined. They can be very sensitive at times, but hesitate to display it. Women have always been the matriarchs of society in all cultures, and they've proven to be much cleverer than men are if they choose to be. In my estimation, women are smarter and emotionally more powerful than men. Women may suffer more depressions, but men commit more suicide.

Women often have the ability to influence a man. They raise our children and the man nods his head to her to indicate his approval or disapproval. The mother fosters music lessons and anything intellectual, while the dad wants their sons to be the best baseball or football player. It is not often that the father encourages his son to be a ballet dancer. A general in the army is fine, as is a run for the presidency. "My son the doctor" is not as proudly said as "my son is earning hundreds of thousands of dollars on Wall Street." In our present Yale Medical School senior class, nearly 50 percent of the class is women. More men are rushing to work on Wall Street!

The best way I can illuminate the difference between men and women came from a patient of mine named Emily, who then became Edwin. Emily was a small woman, not particularly attractive, sad-looking but pleasant, and feminine. She had a small delicate build. She was shy, withdrawn, and worked as a seamstress in New Haven.

Unbeknownst to me, Emily underwent a sex change operation, and when she consulted me I did not recognize her. She now called herself Edwin; her breasts were gone and she spoke in a deep, imperious voice.

"You don't know who I am," she said, "I was a patient of yours and I was Emily, the shy, scared seamstress."

Edwin now smoked two packs of cigarettes per day, drank six to eight ounces of vodka each day, and had muscles. Edwin came to me because he needed someone to give him his weekly testosterone shot. Emily had a hysterectomy and her ovaries removed. I referred him to a family physician, and three years later, I was called in to see Edwin because he had just had a massive heart attack. He had a bypass operation, and when he woke up, he was angry and aggrieved. He continued to smoke and became offensive when the doctors preached a prohibition on smoking. Five years later, Edwin died. He had cancer, a stroke, and another heart attack at the age of 47. We attributed his heart problems partly to his large weekly doses of testosterone, which he needed to keep his male physique. What a price some men are willing to pay.

Chapter Three

Male Aging Myths

MYTH #1:

Memory loss is a normal part of aging

"I can't remember peoples' names. When I meet a client, he tells me his name, and a few minutes later I forget it. Sometimes I walk into a room and I forget the reason," Harry lamented to me during an office visit.

"I am afraid I am getting old before my time, the big 'A' if you know what I mean." Harry is 43 years old and works in a tough corporate environment. He fears he is getting Alzheimer's disease.

"Don't write that on my chart, Doc, I know the HMOs come and read the charts. There is no more privacy in our country. If my bosses learn I have memory loss, they will get rid of me."

Harry was right on all his assumptions, except the myth that aging causes severe memory loss. Harry passed all his mental memory tests with flying colors. Once he learned to concentrate more on peoples' names and repeat them several times during a conversation, he was able to retain their names.

I told Harry that some people are too boring and unimportant for him to remember their names.

Short-term memory loss can sometimes be an initial symptom of a brain degeneration disease, such as Alzheimer's disease or the consequences of numerous medical conditions, medications, and depressions long before short-term memory loss sets in.

A good memory is a God-given asset. We inherit smart brains and good memories if our genes happened to line themselves up to be brainy. We can improve our memories up to a certain point. It all has to do with how many nerve cells (called neurons) we have in the brain. Some persons are blessed with billions of neurons located in the memory part of the brain (called the hippocampus). Scientists have estimated the number of neurons to be from two billion to twenty billion. By the age of 26 onward, we tend to lose neurons. By the age of 90, it has been estimated we have lost approximately 60 percent or more of cells from the entire brain, but not from the critical memory area called the hippocampus. Illnesses such as Alzheimer's disease cause brain loss in the memory area.

Infections, head injuries, and a condition called anoxia, which means that not enough oxygen arrives to the brain, cause neurons to retract like the dead branches of a tree.

A study performed by Dr. Marian Diamond, a neuropathologist, shows that rats deprived of exercise and sensory stimulation have an increased death of nerve cells.

Nerve cells once destroyed will not regenerate and nerve cells cannot be replaced. An adult brain does not make new nerve cells. This discovery was the result of carefully designed studies on monkey brains by Dr. Pasko Rakiv, a renowned neuropathologist at Yale University. In 1985, Dr. Rakiv reported that no new neurons formed in the adult monkey's brain; this became the unchallenged view until October 1999. A new report on monkey brains by Princeton scientists found hundreds of thousands of new neurons arrive each day in the cerebral cortex, where higher intellectual functions are centered. This exciting new concept, discovered by Dr. Elizabeth Gould and Dr. Charles G. Gross, was reported in the *Journal of Science* in October 1999. These noted scholars studied brains of macaque monkeys and watched them produce new brain cells that migrate and develop as they reach the outer core of the cortex (the hippocampus), and make connections with other neurons. This study still has to be confirmed in adult humans.

This new concept, that if brain cells that were destroyed now can be regrown, will revolutionize our entire perception of what the brain is capable of doing. Not only will we be able to make new brain cells, even increase our intelligence, but treat strokes and the worst degenerative disease of our time: Alzheimer's disease. This new notion is like learning for the first time the earth is round and not flat and we won't fall off at its periphery!

"Old age must be resisted and its deficiencies supplied by taking pains. We must fight it as we do disease," said Cicero. I might add that aging is not an illness, but illness causes premature aging. Since recorded times men have been looking for means to prolong life, increase sexual abilities, and save their memories—all of which I will discuss in another chapter.

Men tend to lie to themselves and to others, and ignore symptoms, especially when it comes to memory loss. Two patients of mine, separated by twenty years of practice, come to mind.

Ernie is a nice man who received the Silver Star in the Korean War for saving his squad of five men. He then worked as a supervisor for a large food store chain. His wife was an intelligent woman, a teacher in high school, and she was always vigilant regarding the health of her husband. She knew the color of his stools and urine, and was sensitive to his every-third-day sexual need to have an orgasm. She inspected his body, just like apes do to each other. But when Ernie no longer wanted to have sex and slept more than usual, she decided there was another woman. Each day when he came home from work she sniffed his body, kissed his lips passion-ately, and inspected his clothes and underclothes—yet she found no trace of infidelity.

Not only did Ernie sleep more hours but also he acted duller than usual. His memory was always limited as well as his intellectual capacities, but now he "seemed distracted, out of it, as if someone has drugged him." She watched him sleep and observed him as if he were under a microscope. He had no fever, his appetite began to fail, he lost weight, and even though she increased his daily dosage of natural foods and pills, it did not help. Sweet, loving Ernie became impatient, abusive, rude, and ready to strike at his wife over any minor disagreement. She remembered the movie *Dr. Jekyll and Mr. Hyde*; Ernie had become Mr. Hyde. He was always touching and banging his head against the wall, grinning, "because it makes me feel better."

Ernie one morning got out of bed and walked as if he was on the deck of a ship in a storm. His body was angled to the right so as to keep his balance in check. When his wife saw him come into the breakfast room walking like a drunken sailor, she rushed him to my office. His general examination was normal but he walked with glaring eyes tilted to the right and he was abusive, angry, and had no idea where he was. He forgot my name after ten years of seeing him for yearly physicals. He did not know the name of his children, his address, the year, or who was president of the United States.

We admitted him to Yale New Haven Hospital before the days of CAT scans and MRIs and, because he was hallucinating, a psychiatrist saw him and gave him the diagnosis of acute psychosis of a cause to be determined. Drugs and alcohol were ruled out as the cause. We performed a spinal tap and the spinal fluid was indicative of an infection, but he had no fever. Our teacher, Dr. Paul Beeson, the chief of medicine taught us to look for tuberculosis meningitis; we did, and that was Ernie's diagnosis. He was treated and cured from his memory loss and hallucinations.

Another patient of mine, a professional man, began to lose his memory after a "bad cold." His wife insisted that I see him because he was also drinking too much. He was having episodes of hallucinations and paranoid behavior, which I discovered after I asked him, "Do you ever awake at night and hear voices, or see anything crawling on the ceiling?" He smiled and said, "How did you know, doctor?" I answered, "Well, you and I were trained in the same place." His spinal tap also showed tuberculosis meningitis and the good man was cured—but he still, to this day, doesn't recall that he was admitted to Yale New Haven Hospital.

Roger was 62 when his wife died of lung cancer. He prepared for her death for one year after the doctors told him his wife's cancer had spread to her brain. Every one of his friends was pleased that Roger took it so well and went on with his life. He refused to meet another woman as he said, "I had one wonderful life with my wife, a marvelous marriage, and I don't need another." He lived alone and continued working as a land surveyor. He saw his physician once a year for a checkup and his doctor noticed the neat, well-groomed man began to look slovenly. His shoes used to be shined to a sparkling military style, he was previously clean shaven, and wore a stiff starched, white button-down shirt. A dirty-looking outfit now replaced it. He now had the appearance of someone who had just woken up and climbed out of bed. His children noticed the change and his oldest daughter took Roger to the doctor. As it turned out, Roger was losing his memory and the doctor told the daughter he might be suffering from early Alzheimer's. As there really were no definitive tests for Alzheimer's disease, it was not easy to confirm the diagnosis. The doctor was a shrewd diagnostician and knew from experience that patients with Alzheimer's disease, who knew they were losing their memory, often fabricate answers. Like one of my former patients who was president of a bank, when asked, "Who is president of the United States," replied, "You know, the same old guy; why bother me with such a silly question?"

Roger answered, "I don't know and I don't care . . . wait a minute, it is President Nixon, isn't it? I am too tired to think." It turned out Roger was suffering from a delayed severe depression, which was treated with antidepressants, and his memory and well-being returned.

Often depression can masquerade as Alzheimer's disease and many times it is difficult to separate the two. Sometimes only a therapeutic trial of antidepressants can differentiate between the two conditions.

If your spouse, or significant other, is showing signs of memory loss, don't chalk it up to aging. Take him to a good diagnostician who will spend the time to take a thorough history and be prepared to fight with the HMO if more sophisticated tests are needed.

Here is the list of basic tests the doctor should order: CBC, blood sugar, BUN, creatinine, liver profile, thyroid tests, sedimentation rate, lipid profile, an MRI of the brain, a thorough heart examination to rule out valve and muscle heart problems, a urine test, and a rectal examination. A neurologist also should be consulted.

MYTH #2:
The cardiovascular system gets weaker with age

It is a myth, providing significant irreversible pathological changes did not happen at some point in the past. There are, however, normal changes that do occur with aging. The blood vessels lose their glittering smoothness and elasticity. These vascular system changes cause blood pressure to rise—the systolic (upper reading) and the lower diastolic. In many cases this may require medical treatment for high blood pressure (hypertension). The cells of the muscle of the heart (called the myoctes), decrease in number and the heart thickens at a rate of 1 percent per year. A weaker tissue called fibrous tissue normally replaces the heart muscle. In some subjects, the resting heart rates decrease. In spite of these normal aging changes, the function of the heart remains normal at rest. The male who does not exercise reduces a normal response to exercise—the ability for the heart to contract and pour out blood to all the organs (or in physiological terms, the heart reserve is poor).

Go on a six-month exercise-training program and your heart begins to work as an efficient engine. The decline of heart function is halted and reversed, and you will prolong your life. Of course, always consult a physician to get clearance on how much and what kind of exercise is safe. No matter what medical condition is present, exercise can improve that illness if conducted judiciously.

The major reasons for men not wanting to exercise are joint pain and muscle pain, and plain laziness. For those men who have knee and ankle pain due to arthritic and degenerative changes, exercise is still possible if the men return to their fetal environment: water. "But I can't swim," said the man to his wife. Exercise can be performed in any pool, lake, or ocean in four feet of water. For instance, performing a breaststroke in the water: twenty strokes at a comfortable pace during a half-hour session, three to four times per week. My own prejudice is to exercise every other day to allow the muscles and bones a rest period. The lucky men who are free of joint problems can go dancing, play tennis, walk, bike, run, or join a health club.

The American Heart Association and the American College of Sports Medicine have guidelines for weight training and aerobic programs. In my practice, patients who follow these guidelines do very well, but the majority quit after a few years. Many have spent thousands of dollars to set up their own personal gym in the basement, which in a few years or less becomes their own personal dust collector.

The recommendation from the College of Sports Medicine and cardiologists is that the duration of one session should be less than one hour and should be based on one's heart rate. For example, a previously sedentary person should try to achieve 30 to 40 percent of desired heart rate for that age, as found in the American Heart Association exercise table, for 15–20 minutes, 3–5 times a week for several weeks.

If the subject tolerates it, then it can be increased by five minutes every two weeks until 50 to 70 percent of the age-adjusted heart rate is achieved.

Exercise reduces the blood pressure and is one of the keys to successful aging and freedom from heart disease and strokes. Senior men, aged 71 to 93, who walked two miles a day had half the risk of a heart attack according to a study of 2,678 men from a Honolulu Heart Program, reported in the journal *Circulation*.

In reality, exercise is boring and doomed to failure if the male does not do something he enjoys, or if his wife doesn't show interest. Lucky is the man who plays tennis, or loves swimming.

The best exercise prescription that I can recommend is walking a mile or two per day, or dancing! Most people don't like exercise and do not have the time to follow all those recommendations by the health professionals. I have patients who go square dancing three times per week or disco dancing at home for twenty minutes. Using stairs instead of elevators is also an excellent form of hidden exercise.

During the basketball, football, or baseball season, the male is content to sit on the couch, drink beer and "just relax after a tough day." You can't take that away from them, but they can compromise and do 20 to 30 minutes of exercise before sitting and watching the game.

If you play golf, don't use a cart. Walk and carry your own golf bag.

MYTH #3:

All men lose their libido when they reach a certain age

A seventy-five-year-old man consulted his doctor.

"I just married a twenty-eight-year-old woman. I have a problem, Doc."

"You do have a problem."

"You don't understand, doctor, it's not that. I can't remember her name."

Men lose their libido and become impotent for many reasons. Then the spouse may lose her sexual interest. "He can't do it anymore, so I don't miss it," and a vicious circle ensues.

A man should be able to sustain an active, satisfying sex life well into his eighties and beyond. Problems in the bedroom are more likely due to illness or trouble in his relationship.

What amazes me is how so many men with multiple medical problems still remain active sexually. One patient of mine is 87 and complained to me that he is slowing down; he can only make love to his wife three times a week. Another widower, also 87 years old, is upset because in the senior housing where he lives he can't find a woman who will have sex with him. He has no erection problems.

S.P. is six feet tall, 68 years old, suffering from cancer of the larynx (from smoking), heart disease, vascular disease, emphysema, kidney failure, and arthritis. Casually, I asked this man if he has erectile dysfunction. He replied, "You mean like Mr. Dole?"

"Yes, the way it is alleged," I answered.

"No sir, that ain't one of my problems," he said proudly as I looked on, perplexed. With all those other medical problems, he still managed to lead a healthy sex life.

Some younger men in their thirties, forties, and fifties, lose their libido because of too much stress, drugs, alcohol, and sleeping pills. (See Chapter 7 on Impotence.)

The Massachusetts Male Aging Study, conducted from 1987 to 1989 with 1,700 men, discovered that age was unrelated to satisfactory sex life. This study was conducted in Boston with men between the ages of 40 and 70. They reported a significant decline in sexual desire and intercourse, and the onset of impotence, as they got older. The related causes were depression, cigarette smoking, and repressed expressions of anger. Another study, conducted by the National Health and Social Life Survey in 1992, found a decline in sexual desire beginning at the age of 30! Many men had trouble maintaining an erection as they aged. This survey discovered that sexual dysfunction was due to anxiety about performance, lack of interest, urinary tract problems, poor health, and stress. In my occupation, having seen nearly hundreds of thousands of men over the course of thirty-eight years, I found the main causes of sexual problems to be alcohol, drugs, diabetes, medications, depression, smoking, and bad marriages or relationships—*not* age.

MYTH #4:
Older men don't need as much sleep as they did when they were younger

This is nonsense. We all need uninterrupted sleep whether we are old or young, but each man has different sleep patterns. Some of my lawyer and doctor friends are up before dawn and go to bed early and need only five to six hours; other men need eight to ten hours. Sleep disturbance can be a signal of serious disease.

Insomnia is one of the most common complaints physicians receive, second only to pain. According to a 1984 report by the National Institute of Mental Health, insomnia affects 35 percent of our American population and it costs the American public $100 billion annually in medical expenses. It can be a symptom of cardiac, pulmonary, metabolic, muscoloskeletal, or psychiatric disorders. Interestingly, we sleep 25 percent less than our forebears did one-hundred years ago.

A diagnosis of insomnia is not as simple as it would appear at first glance. Some persons need little sleep and awake alert and rested. Others may need ten hours but only get eight hours; they become sleep deprived and could be considered as suffering from insomnia. Night shift workers sleep eight hours less each week than day workers. Some patients have told me that they have not slept at all in months, even years. Objective sleep evaluation of these patients has shown that they have slept for hours yet they will vehemently deny that they have slept.

Insomnia means the person has not had a sufficient amount of sleep, and the following morning the person wakes up tired and not refreshed. Their reflexes may be altered, physical endurance diminished, memory loss can occur, and they can be a danger to themselves or to the public while driving a car or operating heavy machinery. Major industrial accidents, such as the Chernobyl explosion, the Exxon Valdez spill, and the Challenger disaster, have been officially attributed to excessive daytime sleepiness. In the United States annually, it has been estimated that 100,000 drivers fall asleep at the wheel, resulting in 2,000 deaths.

Lifestyles that include excessive smoking, alcohol consumption, or coffee drinking can cause insomnia in many people. Some subjects are excruciatingly sensitive to caffeine. One of my doctor friends cannot drink even a half-cup of decaffeinated coffee lest he be awake all night. Insomnia can be made worse by trying to solve the sleep disturbance with alcohol.

Less serious conditions, such as restless leg syndrome, are found in about 10 percent of the population at all ages. It is characterized by involuntary movement of the legs with or without numbness at night, which usually interferes with sleep. Neurologists prescribe several medications for the condition, as for example, Klonopin.

Insomnia is not a disease; it is a symptom of a constitutional disorder that can be medical, drug related, or psychiatric. Long-standing insomnia should alert the spouse that a doctor's visit is mandatory.

Excessive daytime sleepiness not caused from sleep deprivation is not related to aging, but can be caused by conditions such as narcolepsy, sleep apnea, sleeping pills, or some rare neurological illness.

Narcolepsy, which means excessive daytime sleepiness, affects 250,000 people in the United States. More than 90 percent of narcolepsy sufferers carry an abnormal gene: HLA type. It occurs more often in young people, and is not a manifestation of aging. People with this disorder can suddenly fall asleep, especially during quiet periods such as when reading, driving a vehicle, during classes, and often watching television.

There was a married intern who was always yawning and falling asleep during many of my lectures. I did not feel insulted, annoyed yes, but not insulted. You see, internship is one of the most grueling and difficult periods in the process of becoming a doctor. It requires unusual physical and mental endurance and self-sacrifice that few could endure. Thirty-six hours without sleep is a good reason to fall asleep during my teaching lectures; I suspect there may be other reasons as well.

But this intern fell asleep during the day, even if he did not work for thirty-six hours. His beautiful wife reported to me that he has the most frightening dreams after they have sex; he would also sleepwalk, and he was always falling asleep during the day (sometimes even during sex). Once he walked naked out of their apartment, sleepwalking, and she screamed after him. He hallucinated and became violent, and that was when she urged him to see a diagnostician. I suspected narcolepsy and referred him to a sleep clinic and a neurologist. The latter successfully treated him with medication (modafinil). Now he is finishing his residency training, he's alert, and a superior medical doctor, though he still falls asleep during my lectures!

Sleep apnea is currently a fashionable diagnosis in men who snore. This does not mean that every patient who snores has sleep apnea syndrome, but snoring accompanied with behavioral changes during the day, memory loss, disorientation, and the continual desire for sleep is indicative of this syndrome.

The diagnosis can be made by the spouse and verified in a sleep clinic.

Shirley and Michael came to my office feeling distraught. Shirley had a black eye and bruises on her face. This happily married couple's relationship began to deteriorate in the past year and she became a "chronic wreck," as she described herself. "All he does is complain to me about his dizzy spells, back pain, his tongue burning, always being tired, yawning, and never wants to have sex. Every night he snores so loud the neighbors complain. Last night my snoring husband starts swinging at me. He hit me in the eye and face, which you can see. He also bruised my breast, which I don't need to show you, and his breath is disgusting. Then all of a sudden he stops breathing, and lies there like a dead mackerel."

Sleep apnea is not part of aging but most often is caused by obstruction of the upper respiratory tract. Michael was diagnosed by the ear-nose-throat doctor to have chronic nasal obstruction from a polyp, and in addition, an abnormality of his larynx that caused it to close at night, resulting in sleep apnea. Surgery was performed for the removal of the polyp and his deviated septum was fixed. Early in his stay in the hospital it was discovered that his oxygen level was below normal; after surgery it was normal. The snoring stopped, the fatigue left, and there were no more night punches to Shirley's face.

Some authors have called this "Ondine's curse," which refers to the revenge that Ondine, a river nymph, took upon the nefarious mortals who deceived her. The punishment was that when they fell asleep, they would stop breathing and die.

This condition, when left untreated, can cause heart failure, memory loss, and hypertension.

All these disorders can be diagnosed in a sleep clinic with tests such as the polysomnogram (which records sleep patterns), and the Multiple Sleep Latency Test (which records eye movements during sleep).

Here are some basic rules to encourage restful sleep: avoid nicotine, alcohol, and caffeine at bedtime; decrease excessive time in bed; avoid late-night dinners; follow a regular pattern of sleep; avoid doing busy work at bedtime (such as balancing your checkbook); don't watch TV in bed; and if you do wake up in the middle of the night, don't linger in bed; get up and read until you get tired, then return to bed. The bed should be a reflex for going to sleep. Try not to nap during the day, and, if all else fails, consult a physician.

Chapter Four

Choosing the Right Doctor

MOST MEN DON'T REALLY CARE too much for doctor visits. One recent AMA survey found that one out of three men didn't have a regular doctor, as compared to one out of five women. One out of five men said they would seek medical care if sick, but would wait at least three days or a week. One out of four men did not see a doctor in years. One of my colleagues admitted to me that he had not seen a doctor in twenty years or more.

On a hiking trip in the Tetons I met a sprightly elderly man and his wife who were both in their eighties. They readily kept up the pace of climbing up the breathtaking hills and valleys with the other hikers, who were twenty and thirty years younger.

I asked the husband, "What is your secret for your long life?" He answered instantly, "I had the right doctor—that is the most important person in your life; choose the wrong doctor and your life will be shortened. If you need a lawyer and he is a dummy—and there are plenty of those lurking around—he, too, can ruin your life."

Imagine if you picked a doctor who carved his initials onto a patient, like Allen Zarkin did to a woman at the Beth Israel

Medical Center in New York after performing a successful cae-sarean operation. Or you could have picked Dr. Michael Swango, who was accused of murdering at least thirty-five patients in an eighteen-year career, and was still allowed to practice medicine! Additionally, Dr. Swango had enjoyed an excellent reputation.

How about the notorious Dr. Max Jacobsen in New York who had a sterling practice among the rich and famous, includ-ing President John Kennedy and lyricist Alan Jay Lerner? Dr. Jacobsen injected Dexadrine in hundreds upon hundreds of patients for many years until his license was revoked. The rich and famous sought him out for their medical care because "he had a great reputation," and Dexedrine gave them more endurance, increased alertness, and rid them of fatigue. Another notable example of choosing the "wrong" doctor was Paul Niehas, who gave his "magical" injections (extracts from animal organs) to people like Bernard Baruch, Gloria Swanson, Somerset Maugham, and Pope Pius XII. The doctor called it "cellular therapy". Then there was Dr. Anna Aslan from Romania who gave secret injections called Gerovital, a mon-amine oxidase (MAO) inhibitor, to Charles de Gaulle, Ho Chi Minh, Marlene Dietrich, and Nikita Kruschev. All these injec-tions were alleged to increase strength, improve memory, delay aging, and make the person more vital. There is no evidence that those injections actually helped!

Today, charlatans run rampant throughout the world; they are fostered by the rich, who can afford to search for the non-existent secrets of the fountain of youth. This is an age-old problem. Just read the Edmund Rostand novel, *Doctor Knock*, which was written in the early nineteenth century. It showed how a layman was able to induce thousands of sick people to come to his office to get "the cure" by using huckster techniques, much like what the HMOs do to induce the poor old-sters to join. "We have the best medical program suited for you," they advertise, until you need their help outside of their "catered plan".

Recently, the Supreme Court denied a patient, injured by the actions of her HMO, the ability to sue.

Each time I am invited to dinner with a wealthy family it makes me cringe how some of them boast of their great heal-ers who, in reality, are not so great, even quite dangerous in some cases.

During my internship days in New York we had labels for the different surgeons who arrived at the hospital. One par-ticular buffoon comes readily to mind; we called him "Dr. X," the killer who invariably complained in the operating room that he got the worst cases, and thus he had the worst out-come. Yet patients continued lining up to be operated on by Dr. X. At that time (1960) no one complained.

"The operation was a success but the patient died." I have heard that too many times. As a matter of fact, it was just this insensitive statement that triggered me to write a book enti-tled *Examine Your Doctor*, which did not ingratiate me at all with my colleagues. With the new medical system, the doctor-patient relationship has gone by the wayside.

One of my patients, having come to me for 30 years, was forced to leave my practice because he switched insurance. I was listed as a cardiologist, but not a primary care physician, and they would not pay for any visits to me unless he first got a primary care physician to refer him to me. The referral sys-tem has many flaws. If his primary care physician plays golf with one of his cardiologist friends, he certainly would not refer this patient back to me. This HMO had solicited an eld-erly patient; the gentleman really did not understand the new medical system. I tell this story to illustrate that today most people have little choice of which physician or hospital to go to. "The doctor has to be on the plan." It is a constant battle for me if I want to refer a patient outside his HMO plan because I feel for a particular condition; a doctor with greater expertise would serve the patient better. But he has no choice to go outside his plan if he is a middle-class American worker with limited income.

It is a very difficult thing to pick one doctor, much less a second doctor. Prior to the HMO revolution most doctors went to their doctor of choice and there was no such thing as ever receiving a bill. At Christmas time, the doctor treated by his colleague received a good bottle of brandy. Professional courtesy was the code of the day. Today, doctors rely on insurance, but still are very cautious!

If you are shopping for a good surgeon for your husband, it is one of the most important decisions you'll ever make. Your family doctor is the one to turn to for the best advice. You want someone who is affiliated with a reputable hospital. You want someone with proper training, and with board certification. Ideally, the surgeon should have loads of experience operating on the specific problem. Even then you need a little luck, no matter how rich and famous you are. Take for example the famous artist, Andrew Wardlow, who died at New York Hospital after a common gall bladder operation. Surely he had the best care money can buy.

I recently diagnosed a young man with lung cancer. His New York family urged him to see an excellent surgeon on Park Avenue. The surgeon was a heart surgeon, and he hadn't performed any lung operations in the past five years. "Better see a surgeon who does mostly lung surgery," I told the family.

My fiancée was discovered to have a rare spinal cord tumor meshed in with the spinal cord. An operation not expertly performed would have left the young woman paralyzed. I searched and asked questions to find a surgeon who had performed this operation more than once. One surgeon in New York said to me, "No problem, bring her here, I can take care of this." I checked with some of my colleagues and found out he had a great reputation but poor surgical results. Much to my pleasure, the best neurosurgeon for this rare tumor was in New Haven and he performed a successful operation on my fiancée. I am telling you this true tale to demonstrate to you that even doctors have the same problem as the rest of the world in choosing the right doctor. As one of my colleagues said to me, "The doctor you get will depend on if he's available, 'on call' that day. Today solo practitioners are dinosaurs—groups dominate the practice of medicine."

Usually, the persons who really know the skills of the surgeon are the anesthesiologists, the residents, and the operating nurses at the hospital who operate with the surgeon. They know the real skills of the operator, but they still keep to the silence code because they will never get a residency in surgery if they blow the whistle on a senior surgeon whose skills have become less effective.

Useful information can be found from the medical association, the insurance carrier, or the HMO regarding the credentials of the surgeon, the number of malpractice suits the surgeon has incurred, and whether the medical board has sanctioned him or her. You can also find out if he carries malpractice insurance. If not, the reason may be because he was dropped.

There is a national Practitioner Data Bank, which went into effect in 1990, which is also an excellent source of information about the doctor you choose.

The all-knowing information superhighway can say what it wishes. A doctor's Web page is not necessarily the best source to use when choosing a doctor. "It pays to advertise," is the old Madison Avenue anthem. Doctors now can advertise themselves just the same as Campbell's soup. I recently was "invited" by the *Advocate* newspaper to submit a profile of myself and my practice for a nominal fee. So were dozens of others. *Who's Who in America* is also a source of information for the public. Being invited to be listed in *Who's Who* does *not* guarantee a superb physician.

Unfortunately, doctors are not immune to the bad ways of the world. In fact, some studies have stated that 10 percent or more of doctors have some sort of addiction.

The good news is that each medical board has a standing ethics committee, as do all the hospitals and HMOs, which together are out there to try to protect the public from the unscrupulous or unskilled physician. They perform a thorough job to rid the profession of "bad apples."

The lawyers have told me that the best doctors get sued more often than the worst because they have the most difficult cases and will have the highest mortality rates. During a recent malpractice case, the lawyer suddenly went into cardiac arrest. The doctor who was being sued saved the lawyer's life with CPR and, later, the same lawyer, after he was well again took up the same suit against the same doctor. The favorite line of these litigators is, "Don't take this personally, doctor."

Patients used to admire and care for their doctors until recently; doctors now are looked upon with suspicion and they aren't as trusted as before, thanks to the poor PR they have received from the media.

Having an office crammed with patients, and beautifully decorated with Persian rugs, paintings on the wall, and a perfect, smiling receptionist, does not tell us of the quality of medical care. Paul Dudley White, the once famous cardiologist from Boston, had a small Spartan office; he was the doctor to President Eisenhower and was a marvelous teacher and innovator.

Good credentials are important in choosing a doctor for your husband; however, they too can be deceiving. If the doctor is well-known in his field, even a full-time professor, he may be spending most of his time lecturing and traveling to conferences, heading a department and spending one day a week seeing private patients. Choose a doctor who practices medicine and surgery on a full-time basis, and is not the sweetheart of the media, or someone running a business on the side. I have known some busy physicians who are also very successful business people, running convalescent homes or other enterprises.

My own prejudice is to choose a doctor who loves the practice of medicine, is well-educated in his field, is devoted to his patients, and is honest and ethical. A doctor, or a member of his group, should be available twenty-four hours a day, including weekends. If the doctor fails to answer your telephone call, find out the reason. If he or she, or a member of the team, ignores your call, change doctors *tout de suite*.

Medicine is a calling and the majority of practitioners are devoted to their patients in spite of the nefarious HMOs. It is a very hard task to become a physician. We gave up the best young years of our lives, at least ten, to become doctors.

If the doctor is affiliated with an approved hospital, he has to spend a certain number of hours in continued medical education if he wants to keep his privileges. Be sure the doctor you choose is affiliated with the hospital of your choice and is approved by the HMO in which you have enrolled.

I see no point in interviewing a doctor before deciding to use him or her as your primary care physician. If he is on your roster or you see him for a physical, make your own observation and conclusion.

The doctor-patient relationship should be governed by the way he makes you feel. You should feel *better* after you see a doctor, not worse. Even bad news can be given to you with optimism, careful explanations, and any alternatives available. The doctor should make you feel confident and you should not be afraid to ask questions. There are no dumb questions in medicine, only dumb answers. You should not feel that you ought to know the meaning of words when the doctor uses unfamiliar medical terms. If you really don't know what they mean, simply ask. For example, what exactly is a heart attack? Or heart failure? Or arrhythmia? If the doctor is curt in his response, ask him why he is being that way. "Alas, doctor, I know you are famous and excellent, but I really don't understand any of this. I wish I did have a medical education. I realize your time is precious and there are many other patients sicker than I or my husband, but would you mind giving me a little explanation." That is how you should respond. If he is still curt, get another doctor. There are plenty of good doctors around, even on your limited HMO list.

If your husband needs surgery, there is no reason not to ask the doctor some basic questions, such as:

Question: "I know you can understand my fears, but as to the operation you planned, how many open heart operations have you performed?"
Good Response: "At least three a week or more."
Bad Response: He gets insulted.

Question: "What is your death rate from this operation?"
Good Response: "I am proud to tell you I have not had one in recent memory, unless the case was very critical to begin with."
Bad Response: "I don't keep track."

You should expect the surgeon to see you before surgery and after surgery. I don't care how great and famous a surgeon he is, if you contract him to operate on your husband's body and you never see the surgeon before or after the surgery, it should make you indignant. I would not let a surgeon operate on my family or me unless I met and talked to him, unless, of course, it is an emergency situation.

I have known some cases where the patient never saw their heart surgeon until their postoperative visit to the office two weeks later. Likewise, unless an urgent situation arises, if you are going to have angioplasty (balloon or stent) on your heart or leg arteries you should know the operator. Too often, the patient says, "I received a bill from this doctor who claimed he performed the angioplasty, and I never saw him." It may very well be that the patient forgot, but certainly the family should have known him.

"I can't stand that man, his beard smells, and he looks like he just got out of bed, but I know he is a good doctor, even if he behaves like some down-on-his-heels character. I still go to him." Or another patient laments, "He is the most arrogant son of a bitch I ever met; he is insulting, but I still go to him because he has a terrific reputation."

If you don't like your doctor for whatever reason, you don't have to keep seeing him, no matter how great he is alleged to be. You still have some choices on your HMO list.

Most doctors today are much more knowledgeable and more patient-oriented than in the past because they can no longer hide beyond the mystique of medicine.

They are under constant scrutiny by the insurance companies, hospitals, emergency room facilities, the Internet, the federal and state government, and lawyers. Information on all new forms of treatment appears in newspapers even before they are published in medical journals.

Doctors today have to accumulate a certain number of hours each year attending medical courses in order to become recertified and keep their hospital privileges. This is called CME, or certified medical education. Connecticut requires a minimum of 60 hours per year to maintain hospital privileges, and so do many HMOs.

Finding the right doctor today is in some ways easier than in the past. The HMOs or hospitals won't keep on their list an unqualified doctor who has not fulfilled his or her post-graduate obligations, or who has been repeatedly sued for malpractice. Medical doctors are investigated if they were sanctioned by their peers or investigated by the state grievance board. Some lawyers and doctors call their boards, consisting of both lay and professional people, "Salem Witch Hunters."

Although the patients have a limited choice of whom to choose for their care, they can still get opinions from their friends and relatives on which doctor to choose from their insurance list.

But don't rely on developing a long-enduring relationship as in the past because as you may have already learned, "I like this guy, but my insurance changed, so I have to pick another one."

Everyone wants the ideal physician: He has to be kind, devoted, well-trained, and a good listener. He is someone who doesn't rush, who is humble, thorough, and is up-to-date on the best treatment. The ideal doctor is one that readily suggests second opinions, refers to experts when needed, is caring, answers phone calls, and sets appointments promptly —you won't have to wait six weeks or more.

He doesn't just have a nine-to-five practice—he makes himself available at your convenience, and he doesn't simply rely on his physician's assistant for your monthly checkups.

As I tell my staff and students, when you leave the office you should feel better, not worse. Even bad news can sound optimistic. That is the real art of medicine.

Group practice is the norm today, and you will get the doctor who is on call for the night even during the day. With multiple office sites you might have to go another office depending where Doctor Y is placed that day.

All in all, this does not detract from excellent care, even if the doctor practices in a barn.

Once you have chosen the doctor from your insurance list, and received good recommendations from your family and friends, you can check on their credentials. If possible, have your spouse come with you on the first visit and help to make the decision if that doctor is the one you can trust. If not, chose another one from your list.

But doctors have no choice about those who come under their care. They have to treat each person with the same manner and thoroughness, regardless of color, sex, or how obnoxious they are. Some patients have the audacity to be rude, arrive not having bathed for days or even weeks, smelling so bad that the nurse staff can barely go near them. Some cough in our face with no regard to our health. One patient, now deceased, lived with twenty dogs in a small apartment. He never bathed and, once, when he was hospitalized, the nursing staff had to peel the dirt off his body before anyone could examine him. He was not a street person, but a rich, selfish old man. We have to respond on a Saturday night if the patient calls because he or she has a dripping nose. In some ways doctors are like a public utility that can be used any time.

Chapter Five

What Women Should Know About the Prostate

SOL IS A WONDERFUL HUSBAND. He's 63 years old, round as a gourd, a professor of linguistics with three grandchildren, and has been married for thirty loving years. His wife, Thelma, not once complained about her husband's habits, except one.

For two years, Solly, as she called him, interrupted her sleep because he climbed out of the bed, bumped into the night table, shook the bed, and woke up Thelma as he went to the bathroom adjacent to the bedroom, and urinated (grunting and moaning like a cow in labor). Twice a night, without fail, once at one in the morning and again at four in the morning, he engaged in these disruptive toilet visits.

Thelma a Phi Beta Kappa scholar, had read that the prostate gland enlarges and sometimes entirely shuts off the flow of urine, as men hit their prime of life. She read how Benjamin Franklin devised his own tube to place into his bladder, and how "Diamond Jim" Brady, the gambler, had one of the first prostate operations—done by Dr. Hugh Young in 1912. This same doctor operated on Woodrow Wilson.

Thelma also read that a spiky plant called Saw Palmetto helps the prostate gland function. It did not do much for

Sol, and his wife finally got him to see his family doctor, Hugh, who found Sol's prostate the size of a large walnut. She had read that the normal size was that of a small walnut.

Although she knew every inch of her husband's body, she had no idea where the prostate resides or what it does. She did research and found out the location of this elusive gland and its function.

This gland lies innocently, snugly behind the pubis and surrounds the urethra; behind it lies the rectum, in front of the pubis bone. Medical access to this gland is via the rectum—hopefully, by an educated finger or, more cruelly, through the penis.

As the prostate enlarges, it presses on the outlet of the urinary bladder and causes symptoms like Sol's. Sometimes it can shut the flow of urine off, and severe, excruciating pain occurs, pain that can only be relieved by passing a catheter through the penis and pushed past the obstruction, and finally into the bladder. A British parish minister once said, "Oh Lord, take me not through my kidney," when his urine flow ceased from his enlarged prostate as he reeled in pain.

The Bedouins (Arab nomads) rarely develop prostate enlargement because their prostates atrophy from horseback and camel riding.

Sol had a PSA (prostate-specific antigen) blood test taken for prostate cancer. His test was normal. Because Thelma insisted, he saw a urologist who confirmed the diagnosis of benign enlargement of the prostate gland, called BPH (benign prostate hyperplasia).

Most men, 90 percent of us, experience prostate enlargement. One woman patient asked me if women get symptoms of enlarged prostate. I explained to her that only men have this nefarious organ. Unfortunately, she was suffering from urinary incontinence, as was her husband.

Sol's symptom of urinating every three hours at night had increased to every two hours. This condition is called "nocturia"—a slow stream and incomplete emptying of the bladder, followed by a second whirl to urinate minutes later. It is due to the enlarged prostate preventing the emptying of the bladder. Sol, in order not to insult the olfactory sensitivity of his loving Thelma, kept a tissue handy to wipe his penis of any lingering residual urine, which stains the underclothing and eventually makes a patient malodorous.

The urologists' recommendation, universally held, is to try a drug such as finasteride, which can shrink the prostate by as much as 20 percent and reduce the horror of suddenly not being able to urinate at all because of acute obstruction.

I remember when, on many nights, I witnessed the excruciating pain of certain male patients lying in agony because they could not pass urine. Their blood pressure rose and the heart rate increased. In one or two incidences, I have witnessed an elderly man develop a stroke or a heart attack. Trying desperately to pass a urinary catheter into a shrunken penis at four in the morning, while I was an intern, will remain fixed in my brain. The poor patient screamed from the pain as I tried to pass the catheter—and finally a urologist arrived hours later to do the job.

Today, miracle drugs such as tamulosin HCL (Flomax), or so many others, usually help restore the flow of urine to some acceptable degree.

Sol was given tamulosin, which did shrink the prostate gland some; his nightly runs to the toilet decreased and did not interfere with his biweekly sex life.

Other medications a man can try are alpha-blockers; these

do not result in shrinkage of the prostate gland but, rather, they relax the internal sphincter at the bladder neck and prostate. Drugs such as terazonin (Hytrin) and doxazosin (Cardura) are alpha-blockers, but they have their side effects by causing dizzy spells as they lower the blood pressure. Some doctors use these drugs to control elevated blood pressure and urinary problems.

If medications fail and your man is still suffering from prostatism (inability to urinate), surgery for very large prostates may be necessary, or perhaps laser treatment (microwave hyperthermia). There are various other procedures that may be of some value, but only a urologist can advise you on them.

Prevention is the goal and the art of medicine. We know if you don't smoke, keep your weight down, drink in moderation, exercise, have a good outlook on life, a sense of humor, lots of love, enjoy your work, carry as little anger in your heart as possible, and have a good doctor, you should live long—and well!

For men, heart attack, strokes, lung cancer, cancer of the colon, prostate cancer, blood cancers, HIV infections, and trauma are the most common reasons for death.

Cancer of the prostate will eventually show up in 80 percent of us. During my medical school training when we performed an autopsy on patients who died of heart attacks, strokes, and other causes, we found that most men after 70 years old had cancer of the prostate. The cancer did not spread to other organs, and the men did not die of prostate cancer.

In 1999, an estimated 179,300 new cases of prostate cancer were reported; 37,000 American men are expected to die of prostate cancer each year. Most prostate cancers are diagnosed in men 65 years or older. The median age at death from prostate cancer is 78. Mortality among black men from prostate cancer is twice that of white men. Researchers are busily trying to find the reason for this large discrepancy.

The PSA test is a fairly reliable test to detect prostate cancer. This simple blood test must be combined with a rectal examination. As much as 20 percent of significant prostate cancers may record PSA below 4.0 ng/ml (normal up to 4.0). The experienced clinician was able to detect cancer of the prostate by a simple rectal examination for many generations before the PSA test came on the scene.

"I urge everyone to get a PSA test," so said Mayor Rudy Giuliani of New York after his cancer was discovered. Joe Torre, the New York Yankees' manager, told Mayor Guiliani of his experience with PSA testing and the treatment of his prostate cancer.

Yet even though we now have a test to find early cancer of the prostate, there is a great deal of controversy emerging on the value of universal testing of men over the age of forty. The reason is because finding an elevated PSA usually leads to a sonar examination of the prostate and then a biopsy of the gland, which often is normal or at least minimally present. Some men have chosen not to treat early cancer of the prostate as, in many instances, it is slow growing and never leaves its enclosure to spread.

In the near future we can look forward to more precise tests for prostate cancer. They will determine who should have a biopsy and how aggressive the treatment should be.

Urologists use the Gleason score to determine the extent of the presence of the cancer and the best treatment available, which include hormonal, radiation, and surgery. Surgery can leave the man impotent and incontinent. It is beyond the scope of this book to discuss the controversial issues on the best treatment of cancer of the prostate. The spouse's job is to urge her husband to seek expert advice and a second opinion on the best course of treatment, just as Mayor Guiliani has done by getting advice from different doctors.

In summary, I do feel strongly that a rectal examination and a PSA be performed once a year on every male once they reach the age of forty or so. If the PSA is high, as might be found in patients with benign prostate enlargement who do not have cancer, it does not take away the value of screening on a yearly basis.

Can men prevent cancer of the prostate? I have always believed that tomatoes are the secret of good health (and not only because I love fresh-grown garden tomatoes, soaked in olive oil, garlic, and pepper). Every morning, as long as I can remember, I have had a tomato and freshly squeezed orange juice.

The good news is that the unspoiled tomato contains lycopene and carotene—that gives the tomato its alluring bright-red color—which reduces the risk of prostate cancer, according to the Fred Hutchinson Research Center in Seattle, Washington. This was reported in the January 5th, 2000, issue of the *Journal of the National Cancer Institute*. Serve vegetables and you will reduce the risk of prostate cancer.

Another study, from the University of California at Los Angeles, discovered that you don't need fresh tomatoes to lower your cancer rate—V8 100% vegetable juice in the can has an even better concentration of lycopene and carotene. Take your choice, but remember that preventive medicine is often as close as your grocer's shelf. I, for one, would much prefer a fresh ripe, juicy deep red tomato, than a can of juice.

Saw palmetto, the herb described earlier in this chapter, helps to shrink the normal prostate glands, but has little or no effect on the glands that are enlarged. It does not prevent cancer of the prostate, but in some patients it may relieve the frequency of urination in those suffering from benign hypertrophy of the prostate.

Chapter Six

The Fingerprints of Impending Medical Disasters

MY FATHER REFUSED to seek medical attention for back pain that troubled him for months. When I begged him to come to New Haven to get checked out, he refused. He said, "What's the matter, son, business too slow?" Three weeks later I received a call from the emergency room of Jamaica Hospital in Queens. My father had collapsed on the street, diagnosed as having a heart attack; he died one hour later. I demanded an autopsy, which revealed that he did not have a heart attack at all. A ruptured blood vessel in his abdomen killed him. If my father had undergone a thorough examination at the time of his complaint, the abdominal aneurysm could have been diagnosed and treated months earlier. This tragedy haunts me to this day, and eventually compelled me to write a book entitled *Examine Your Doctor*.

Back pain is a common complaint among men, and each complaint needs to be thoroughly investigated. In my practice, even with a normal physical examination, I request a CAT scan of the back to be certain that there is no abdominal aneurysm lurking, or a tumor either of the spine or a metastasis to the backbone present.

Most medical disasters do not happen out of the blue. Many serious medical problems begin with seemingly benign symptoms such as back pain.

My tennis partner, during one of our usual grueling matches, complained of back pain—after he lost the match. We often find excuses for losing: "My game was off today because I did not get enough sleep," "I did not concentrate," etc. He consulted several doctors including a chiropractor, and when he began to lose weight, cancer of the pancreas was discovered. He died eight months later in his home.

THE NEW EPIDEMIC THAT THE SPOUSE SEES EVERY DAY

Years ago, if we survived birth, then we had to survive childhood infections. I remember having all those awful childhood illnesses such as the mumps, chicken pox, measles, scarlet fever, and polio. There was no penicillin when I contracted scarlet fever, and by chance survived the heart and kidney complication that go with it. There was also polio, which was a worldwide epidemic and the only treatment available was Sister Kennedy's massage therapy. Then came the wars, one after another, which killed hundreds of thousands of men. Living beyond the age of 60 was a rare phenomenon. We had little control or chance of avoiding an early death.

Now, more than ever, since the beginning of recorded time, we have so much greater control of our own health. Yet so many men and women do not take advantage of the miracles of medicine. We are living longer (beyond what anyone would have dreamed fifty years ago). In the very near future we can expect to live longer with dignity and better health beyond the age of 100.

Today, the major causes of death we can avoid are AIDS, stroke, heart attack, cancer, lung disease, and drug or alcohol abuse. We do not need a war to cause an early death. We are the ones responsible for so much of our own calamities. Smoking is a prime example of self-destruction.

One of the most glaring examples of self-ruination is the new epidemic of obesity, which is regarded as one of the major causes of heart attacks, high blood pressure, diabetes, strokes, and even cancer. Unfortunately, there are examples in our society where obesity is glorified.

Recently I watched the grotesque, obese King of the Mardi Gras dancing on the streets in New Orleans, and a beauty contest of the "fattest and most beautiful women" in the American Virgin Islands. I also watched the famous Wagnerian opera series called *The Ring* this past spring and listened in awe to the magnificent singing, but at the same time was distressed to see the obesity of some of the female singers who could just barely negotiate their huge bulk across the stage. All was forgiven because their voices seemed to emanate from heaven. Yet I dread to think of what medical disasters may lay before them.

The prevalence of obesity has dramatically increased between 1976–1998. Today, 140 million American adults over the age of 20 are overweight, and 42 million are obese. The irony of it is that the more doctors nag about the dangers of being overweight, the fatter our society gets.

Each year we spend an estimated two billion dollars on weight-loss diets and medications such as "Fen-Phen," which, in some persons, has caused heart ailments that are more perilous than being obese. We have become desensitized to all the propaganda on the dangers of being overweight.

Where does it come from, this frenzy to eat so much? Was it from the time my mother and other mothers urged us to eat as children because the children of China were starving? Who can forget the nutritionists cajoling us to eat the great American breakfast of eggs, bacon, and home fries, and a rich lunch to get through the day, followed by a hearty supper of meat, potatoes, and vegetables topped off with strawberry shortcake? Restaurants serve generous portions of food—one portion is usually enough for two people.

Dr. William Osler, the father of modern American medicine, said in 1928, "When I see a fat person come in the front door, I want to go out the back door."

Today physicians are overwhelmed with overweight patients and many are reluctant to treat them because the failure rate is close to 90 percent! In this HMO climate there is little time allotted for care for the overweight. Doctors do not get rewarded by HMOs or Medicare for spending the time needed to treat overweight and obese patients. There are clinics for weight reduction, but most HMOs will not pay for the visits. One clinic in New Haven requires $70 for the first visit, which most indigent persons cannot afford too easily. The argument posed is, "Well, they can afford to pay that money on food."

How do doctors diagnose obesity? One look is worth a thousand words to give us the subjective estimate measure of a patient's weight. At carnivals you can find a weight expert who will guess your weight within five pounds. But in the scientific world today, the National Health and Nutrition Examination Surveys gave doctors guidelines. Even the Metropolitan Life Insurance Company developed weight tables according to height and age. These are no longer used because they are inaccurate—they measure average weight and ideal weight data gathered from insurance physicals. As many as 20 percent of examiners who reported height and weight actually never measured their subjects.

Today, we use the body mass index (BMI) to classify weight, which is arrived at by a formula. The BMI measures relative weight from height. For example, weight times the height in kilograms, times 1.57 meters squared, will give the doctor the BMI needed to follow your weight loss or gain. Doctors now have simple tables to instantly calculate your BMI.

The *British Journal of Nutrition* submitted tables on measuring fat deposits under the skin by the uses of calipers to measure skin fold thickness.

Waist circumference measurements are also used to determine high risk for diabetes, heart attacks and strokes.

Waist circumferences greater than 40 inches in men and greater than 35 inches in women represent a high and dangerous risk of dying from heart disease. In a recent study, men with waists larger than 36 inches were twice as likely as thinner men to develop colon cancer. Colon cancer kills 23,000 men every year, as reported by Dr. Robert Schoen from the University of Pittsburgh.

HOW DO YOU HELP
YOUR SPOUSE LOSE WEIGHT?

Doctors have failed miserably in their attempts to help patients lose weight. The fat problem is a very sensitive issue for women. Many women refuse to give up smoking, as they fear they will gain weight. For a man it is not so overtly a sensitive issue, but the man will tire of hearing, "You know you should not eat that ice cream," or "You are getting too fat; it's disgusting."

Many times the male may become a closet ice cream or cookie eater—his bad eating habits are practiced outside his home.

What the spouse should say is: "Darling, I love you very much, and I need you. I want you to be at my side as we grow old together and watch our grandchildren grow. Let us work together on your weight problem. I can't think of you becoming ill."

The first step for the spouse is to determine why her mate has gained so much weight. Is he eating more? Has his alcohol intake increased? Has his physical activity decreased? Is he sitting every night and weekend watching TV, or addicted to his computer? Is there a metabolic cause for being overweight? In most cases, being overweight is due to overeating or eating the wrong food, drinking too much alcohol, and getting too little exercise. A thorough physical examination and proper blood testing can find a metabolic cause such as a thyroid or adrenal gland problem.

If all the tests are normal, then comes the difficult part—determining a diet that the man is willing to follow. Based on my thirty-eight years of medical practice I lay out a program for the man—with his spouse present—which caters to his occupation and eating habits. For example, he might be discouraged to have that pastry with his morning coffee break or to skip the evening bedtime snack.

Losing weight has to be a long-term commitment, a change of lifestyle that caused the problem in the first place.

Counting calories is a mainstay of most diet programs. In order to lose one pound you must burn up 3,500 to 4,000 calories. If you use up 1,500 calories per day with ordinary activity and another 500 or so with exercise, while taking in only 1,500 calories you will have a net loss of 500 calories per day. At the end of seven days you will have lost one pound; at the end of a year that will add up to 52 pounds.

"Who has time to exercise," the man says, "to lose those extra calories?" A simple program that will include the wife is dancing! Fifteen minutes of disco dancing can use up anywhere from 100 to 450 calories. Approximately 30 calories are used per minute dancing, depending on the weight of the person. The heavier the person, the more calories they use up. Sexual activity, needless to say, also uses up calories—six calories or more per minute!

I found that the mathematical diets appeal to the male brain, as most men are "counters." We are forever counting our money: how much we earned or lost on a stock. Our pencils and computers are forever making lists of spending and earning and how much money we need to retire.

If it takes five years to lose 40 pounds, that's okay. Rapid weight loss, with various gimmickry diets should not be accomplished in a few months. Proper eating habits with sound reduced caloric intake should be the goal. It has to become a way of life. Too quick weight loss can be dangerous to your health. Allow the metabolic, chemical, and molecular content of your spouse's body to become adjusted to the weight loss. If he loses weight too quickly his friends will wrongly surmise he is suffering from cancer or some other illness, asking, "Are you feeling okay? You look sort of sick."

One of my doctor patients embarked on a high-fat, low-carbohydrate diet to lose weight. He proudly announced to me how he eats steak and bacon and eggs, with no sweets, and lost twenty pounds. He knows quite well that is the best diet to achieve an early death from heart disease, according to the American Heart and American Medical Association. But doctors are not exempt to fall prey to gimmickry diets.

If your spouse wants a safe magic pill to lose weight, it really doesn't exist. The FDA approved "Fen-Phens" which later were found to cause heart problems. In 1997, the drug Sibutramine was introduced. It is supposed to be safe, but in some patients it causes the blood pressure to rise, and an increase of the heart rate. Patients lost four pounds in the first four weeks of treatment, and after six months achieved a 10 percent loss of their body weight. In my practice, I have not prescribed these pills or any other dietary medications. Instead, I have a diet that works very nicely if followed (see Appendix).

HEARTBURN

This is a symptom that has proliferated since men started drinking more martinis, smoking more cigars, eating more spicy food, and swallowing too many aspirin and over-the-counter anti-inflammatory agents. It occurs in 20 percent of the American population.

At one time or another we all have experienced that burning sensation in our chest after a spicy dinner with lots of red wine.

Jim B. had heartburn for years and chewed on antacid pills to relieve his symptoms. He was a jovial, robust, red-cheeked railroad train conductor who "liked his beer and cigarettes." As he left the house for his annual checkup, Molly, his wife, yelled, "Don't forget to tell the doctor about you eating antacid pills all day and about your heartburn."

"Yes, love, I will," he grumbled as he slammed the front door. Now Jim liked his doctor a lot and they both gabbed about the fortunes of the Boston Red Sox as the doctor examined Jim. He had an electrocardiogram and a rectal exam, which Jim hated.

"Go easy on those cigarettes and beer, Jim, and your heartburn will disappear and your belly won't make you look like a six-months-pregnant woman."

He passed his physical with flying colors, he told Molly, "And, can you beat this, my blood pressure is perfect and so is my electrocardiogram."

Two weeks later, a few days before Christmas Eve, Jim went to his Christmas party with the boys and they ordered a delicious large spicy pizza from Gino's and everyone brought a case or two of their favorite beer. That night Jim felt as if his chest and stomach were on fire. While still a little drunk, he jumped out of bed and swallowed a bottle of liquid antacid, which gave him some relief.

"You and your drinking buddies," his wife said half asleep, "you just won't listen or learn."

"I'll see the doc tomorrow, no more beer or pizza or cigarettes for me," he said, "I promise."

In the middle of the night, Molly tried to rouse Jim to make love, but he remained motionless. Big Jim was dead. The autopsy disclosed all the arteries of his heart were blocked and he had had a massive heart attack.

Heartburn is usually caused by the backup of stomach acid into the esophagus—also called reflux—resulting from a condition such as diaphragmatic hernia (sliding stomach), duodenal ulcer, GERD (or gastrointestinal reflux disease), stones in the gallbladder, or spasms of the esophagus (the tube that leads into the stomach beginning in the mouth). The esophagus lies adjacent to the heart, thus clinicians hundreds of years ago called the burning feeling in the chest "heartburn." This symptom too often can fool the patient and the doctor, as it can be almost identical to the symptoms of a heart attack (sudden blockage of the coronary arteries of the heart). Usually heartburn is relieved with antacids and is improved if the patient sits up from a lying position.

R.J. was 55 when he came to the emergency room because he had terrific heartburn after a meal of mussels with a red spicy sauce. The intern on duty administered some antacids and R.J. felt better. The following morning R.J.'s wife urged him to visit his doctor as he still was complaining of some heartburn. An electrocardiogram disclosed R.J. had suffered a heart attack, and his symptom, heartburn, did not result from a spicy meal but from blocked arteries to his heart.

In my first year of medical practice I heard a 58-year-old man in my office complain of heartburn. His electrocardiogram was negative. In those early days we had no coronary care unit or blood tests to determine if a heart attack had occurred—just the electrocardiogram. But because his heartburn was not relieved by antacid, I admitted him to Yale New Haven Hospital, then called Grace New Haven Hospital. It took two days for the electrocardiogram to become abnormal. In those early days we had no clot busters, stress tests, echocardiograms, bypass surgery, pacemakers, or angioplasty, just oxygen and morphine to relieve his pain. We had no idea that aspirin could help stop an attack. He died in the hospital one week later from a ruptured heart muscle.

What should the spouse or partner do if her partner complains of heartburn? She should ask her spouse, "Are you sure, dear, it's from something you ate?" Explain to your spouse there are many causes for heartburn besides smoking, drinking, and eating spicy foods. After you have convinced your man to see a doctor, and if he goes alone, give him a memo to give to the doctor and on it, write:

"Could my heartburn be due to blocked arteries to my heart?"

"Is it from stones in my gallbladder?"

"Is it from gastrointestinal reflux?"

If you go with your spouse and the doctor gives you a "Mr. know-it-all smile," pats you on the back, and says, "Don't worry, it is not necessary to do any tests," change doctors!

The good doctor will arrange for appropriate tests for coronary heart disease if the man has a family history of heart problems, is a smoker, has high cholesterol, or if his heartburn does not follow the usual pattern.

Although heartburn is so often reported by patients, there are about the same number of heart attacks per year as there are cases of heartburn—almost two million. In emergency rooms around the country, too many people are sent out with heartburn, though they are suffering from coronary artery disease. We are educating our young doctors to this calamity, but the HMOs make it difficult to spend the time or allow the doctors to perform the appropriate testing. That is why the *spouse* must take charge and ask the appropriate questions to save the life of her loved one.

At the American College of Cardiology meeting in Anaheim, California, in March 2000, Dr. John G. Canto of the University of Alabama reported that one-third of acute myocardial infarctions did not have the classical chest pain—the hallmark of a heart attack.

PALPITATIONS

Bernard, a nervous type, always felt his heartbeat racing during the day and often during the quiet of the night, when lying on his left side. He consulted many doctors over and over again. All the tests could not detect anything wrong with Bernard's heart, but there was plenty wrong with his mental state. He was suffering from a heart neurosis, one doctor told him, and he had a constant fear he was going to die.

"I feel my heart is doing jumping jacks and sometimes it feels like it is going to stop, and then it races; it's going to jump out of my chest." That is how Bernard described his symptoms.

Bernard got a new girlfriend, who was a nurse, but what he really wanted was a woman doctor to live with him, however; then she could save his life, he reasoned. Ellie, the nurse, was the perfect match for him. She liked skiing, tennis and the opera—and their sex life was very healthy.

One moonlit night, while at Martha's Vineyard, Barnard fell asleep and Ellie placed her head on his chest. She heard his heart pounding and racing just like Bernard had described: fast, slow, and irregular. She woke up her lover in her usual manner and drove him down to the emergency room of the local hospital, and there the EKG taken was normal. But nurse Ellie knew what she heard and told the cardiologist at her hospital about it. This time, instead of the customary 24-hour Holter monitor of the heart, the cardiologist ordered the use of an event monitor to record the heart whenever Bernard felt his heart racing. The results would be transmitted by telephone to a central communication station where it could be reviewed. Lo and behold, one of the heartbeat patterns was classical for ventricular tachycardia, a dangerous rhythm of the heart.

With the proper treatment Bernard no longer had the palpitations. His cardianeurosis was not a neurosis, but a justifiable fear of sudden death. Bernard was so grateful that he decided to give up his single life and marry Nurse Ellie. She had literally saved Bernard's life. This one deadly abnormal rhythm of the heart is often not discovered. These cases of sudden death are sometimes misinterpreted as "death by natural causes."

In the United States at least 250,000 persons die suddenly each year and approximately 100,000 patients have ventricular tachycardia. The most common cause is coronary artery disease.

In the case of Bernard's heart problem no cause was found; we call that idiopathic ventricular tachycardia—a term doctors use when we don't know the cause.

In another case, Raul's wife insisted he consult me because, at the age of 58, she feared he was suffering from hardening of the arteries; he was always complaining of his skipping heart. We performed every cardiac test on him and even used an event monitor, but our team could not find anything wrong with his heart.

On one of his routine visits to my office, as he was describing a fishing trip and as I listened to his heart, its beat suddenly turned irregular. Swiftly, an EKG taken by my medical assistant revealed that Raul was in atrial fibrillation. He was hospitalized, treated, and his blood was thinned out with a medication called Coumadin, which helps prevent strokes.

It is a rather common circumstance that a patient's heart is found to be irregular during a routine office visit. More often than not, the stubborn male docs not tell anyone that his heart is beating strangely and it is discovered only after he has collapsed or, at worst, suddenly died.

Palpitations are called skipped heartbeats, extra heartbeats, or fast heartbeats. They should trigger an investigation to determine the cause and the patient should have it treated if necessary. The spouse should be suspicious of a heart problem if her husband suddenly becomes pale or perspires or looks like he is going to faint. Every partner should learn how to take a pulse. If the pulse is found to be rapid, irregular, or very slow, the emergency squad should be called immediately.

Men in their fifties and older who engage in competitive sports sometimes develop irregular heart rhythms. At the Yale tennis club one fine day, one of the excellent players was volleying with his wife next to my court. She noticed her husband did not look right and insisted they stop volleying. Minutes later he was lying on the ground. My cardiology colleague and I rushed over to him and administered CPR. He had an irregular heartbeat because he had suffered a minor heart attack. In the coronary care unit, he 'fessed up to having skipped heartbeats before, yet he still continued to play tennis. He was a heavy cigarette smoker, and prior to this episode he never had a stress test.

Syncope, or fainting spells, probably occurs at least once in 50 percent of people's lives. In Victorian times fashionable homes had a swooning couch. Young ladies and even young men would get the "vapors," swoon and faint on the wonderfully decorated red velvet couch and be revived by a whiff of some strong astringent or a gentle kiss from a lover. These young people probably were suffering from what we call vago-vagel attacks—a condition where the heart slows and the blood pressure falls, usually because of fright, bad news, or a broken heart.

Men over the age of 50 suffering from diabetes, or who have a history of heart attack, should be brought to the emergency room to rule out another heart attack or an arrhythmia problem like ventricular tachycardia. Other causes the doctor will look for include internal bleeding, embolism (clots traveling to the lungs), and little strokes. Some blood pressure medications, such as beta-blockers, channel blockers, and ACE inhibitors, may lower the blood pressure to an unsatisfactory level.

The condition is called orthostatic hypotension. Doctors should test for orthostatic hypotension—which means the blood pressure falls when the individual stands. More than once when I receive a call from the emergency room that an elderly man on blood pressure medications collapsed, I will ask the resident to have the patient's blood pressure measured while standing for a few minutes. If orthostatic hypotension is the cause, the blood pressure will fall; for example, from a reading of 150 mm systolic to 100, the man may become dizzy and may collapse again. The treatment is to alter the dosage and increase the fluid intake.

Physicians and health workers urge patients to eliminate salt from their diet too often when it is not warranted (unless the patient tends to accumulate water as in congestive heart failure, or suffers from salt-sensitive hypertension, and has a strong family history of hypertension). Low-salt diets can account for weakness and fainting spells, especially in hot, humid weather.

The spouse, if present, or for that matter any other person on the scene, can best describe the events of syncope. Did he just fall? Did he stagger? Become pale? Did you take his pulse? The observer of the syncope event can supply invaluable clues for the reason the person fainted. Doctors need to be more diligent and ask the family detailed questions that can help solve the cause of the collapse.

We all need to be like Sherlock Holmes and look for clues. Sir Arthur Conan Doyle, the author of the Sherlock Holmes stories, was a doctor of medicine. I urge all my medical students to read *The Adventures of Sherlock Holmes* to help learn the deductive process needed so desperately to solve medical mysteries.

STROKES

On April 12, 1945, President Franklin Roosevelt lay dying of a massive cerebral hemorrhage at the age of 63. His blood pressure was recorded at 300/100. Only two months before, Roosevelt had attended the historical meeting at Yalta with Winston Churchill and Joseph Stalin to discuss the end of World War II. Just prior to Roosevelt's death, the president's inner circle reported that the president had brief aberrations in thought process and neurological functions. Some historians say that because the president was having these problems he didn't stand up to Joseph Stalin and that the map of Europe, and the entire world, was adversely changed. Some of the symptoms reported by the president's physician were dizzy spells, numbness of his face, tremors, fleeting moments of forgetfulness, sudden loss of vision in one eye, and weakness of one arm. These are the signs of a prestroke or "little stroke."

The same could be said of President Woodrow Wilson in October 1919, who was in a semi-coma from a stroke while his wife Edith ran the presidency. Likewise, it was known that President Wilson had episodes of little strokes, which we now call transient ischemic attacks (or TIA), while negotiating the Treaty of Versailles, which ended the First World War. Some may say that the disastrous terms agreed upon became one of the causes of World War II. The doctors caring for these presidents were remarkably precise in their diagnoses before the full-blown strokes occurred, without the aid of CAT scans or MRIs. President Richard Nixon also died of a stroke.

Today, the number of strokes is increasing to at least 800,000 per year, and strokes remain the third leading cause of death. Strokes due to arteriosclerosis (hardening of the arteries) occur four times as often in men than in women.

The stroke incidence increases dramatically with age. TIA is the most important symptom as a prelude to a stroke. In a study presented at the 25th International Stroke Conference in 1999 it was shown that a full stroke occurred in one out of four patients within 90 days after a TIA; 50 percent within one year.

Often the man or the primary physician does not recognize the minor symptoms of a TIA. Dr. Larry Goldstein, director of the Duke Center for Cerebrovascular Disease, stated that, "Only 20 percent of patients who think they are having a TIA go to their primary physician, and the private sector does not systematically admit the patients to the hospital or perform appropriate tests." I know from personal experience, if I wish to order a CAT scan on a patient suspected of TIA it becomes a battle of endurance to get approval from the HMO if the patient's symptoms are no longer present.

Symptoms of weakness, numbness on one side of the face, difficult speech, sudden loss of vision, double vision, dizzy spells, fainting, weakness of one extremity that disappears in twenty-four hours, are often indicative of a TIA. By the time the patient sees the doctor the symptoms are gone and the HMO may not approve any of the tests unless a doctor speaks to the head doctor/director. Recently I had to get approval for a CAT scan from the doctor responsible for giving approvals. I asked him, "Doctor, are you a specialist in neurology or internal medicine?" He answered, "No, I am a pediatrician and I am in charge here." Imagine the audacity of the insurance company when I have to get approval for a test that is essential for the patient! I am certain that if the CEO of an HMO, or a member of the White House staff, a member of Congress, or even a mayor, needed essential tests there would not be any delays in getting approval.

As Dr. Claiborne Johnston said: "The acronym TIA should stand for 'Take immediate action'."

Mandel, an accountant, was 69 years old, and suffered from hypertension for years. His blood pressure, taken by his family doctor of thirty years, was controlled by one of the most expensive blood pressure medications that the pharmaceutical companies developed each year. (In spite of newer and newer medications for treatment of hypertension, the stroke incidence has increased dramatically, but death from strokes has decreased.) Mandel's blood pressure was usually around 138/85 when taken after resting for five minutes and several hours after drinking coffee. He also took one aspirin per day (as advertised by the Bayer company on television and as recommended by his doctor) to prevent a heart attack. Many people take aspirin to prevent heart attacks.

His son Benny, an account executive, finally, at the age of 43 found a suitable mate for himself and a wedding was planned in June at a fashionable Southhampton club. Both families invited everyone who was anyone.

Mandel was a happy man but one morning, four weeks before the wedding, he got out of bed feeling lightheaded. He had a headache and his right arm felt numb, and continued to feel numb all day. Since it was tax time, Mandel reasoned it was numb because he overworked preparing tax returns and he simply had overdone it at his gym at the health club in New York—all exacerbated by the stress of the approaching wedding. Oh, such stress! He so wanted to look trim and fit for the wedding.

Mandel consulted his doctor, Morris, who found his blood pressure to be 140/90 and told him to hold off on his weight lifting and jogging. With the wedding only a month away, the doctor said the exercise was only an added stress. A B12 shot was given and twenty-four hours later all symptoms disappeared. No one suspected it was a TIA.

One month later, the wedding occurred. It was a glorious affair with the best champagne and Cuban cigars, which even the Rabbi smoked. As the dancing started, Mandel joined in and he suddenly collapsed on the dance floor. He lay wide-eyed, not able to speak or to move his arms and legs. It was discovered at the hospital that Mandel had a massive cerebral hemorrhage; to this day he remains totally paralyzed.

The tragedy of Mandel might have been averted if all the parties involved, including his wife, were cognizant of the symptoms of a TIA.

There are two types of TIA that lead to two types of stroke. One is called ischemic, which means not enough blood is going to the brain because of blockage of the arteries to the brain; the other is called hemorrhagic, which is a bleeding into the brain, as was the case with Mandel.

Patients who are prone to stroke are those with hypertension, previous heart attacks, abnormal heart rhythms such as atrial fibrillation, high cholesterol, and clotting abnormalities—not to mention heavy smokers and drinkers. Such patients must be made aware that they are prone to TIA, strokes, and obesity. Spouses can be very helpful with this knowledge because men are too often negligent when it comes to their own health.

Mandel's blood pressure was "controlled." So why did he have a stroke? Patients' blood pressure controlled at rest may not be controlled with physical activity. This is called a hypertensive response with exercise. Most strokes occur with a blood pressure reading of 145/90 or higher.

Good blood pressure control means that, at exercise, the blood pressure does not rise above 250 mm, because that could cause a stroke. Ideally, an exercise stress test should be performed for the purpose of recording blood measurements with exercise. Home blood pressure readings with at reliable BP instrument are a good way to control blood pressure. Then the spouse can measure the blood pressure at home, right after her man does vigorous exercise. If the blood pressure rises too fast and too high above 200/100, the doctor can make the proper medication adjustments.

In the United States, 60 million people suffer from hypertension. Too many do not have their blood pressure controlled for many reasons, and many more have no clue that their blood pressure is elevated.

Not long ago, we were taught that the ideal blood pressure was 100 plus your age. It was not an easy task to convince the public and doctors that the ideal blood pressure is 130/75 regardless of age. A recent study, which included the Yale Medical School, discovered that the upper reading, called the systolic, was a crucial determining factor for the cause of stroke. Consistently, readings above 150 mm systolic need to be treated vigorously to achieve the 130/75 goal. Patients many times are responsible for the failure to control their blood pressure. Either they forget to take their medications, or they do not refill their prescriptions; they do not report side effects such as impotence, but just stop their pills—and in America today, many patients cannot afford to pay the exorbitant prices of the medications prescribed. Some go to Canada for a cheaper price.

Headaches may be the outstanding symptom of TIA. Every new headache that the spouse complains of has to be investigated, especially if it awakens him from a sleep, and it is severe or of long duration.

Some basic rules that Jack Klapper, chief of neurology at St. Joseph's Hospital in Denver, suggested for sorting out benign headaches from more serious ones are:

- Severe headaches followed by some neurological sign such as weakness of a leg, numbness, or other deficit, could mean a stroke is impending and is not a migraine headache. Neurological symptoms such as loss of vision or numbness or weakness occur *before* a migraine headache occurs.
- A severe headache—one that the patient has never experienced before—that awakens him in the middle of the night, requires an immediate trip to the emergency room because it could signal a brain hemorrhage.

- Headaches with accompanying mental changes could signal a subdural brain hemorrhage, or an infection, or tumors.
- Headaches that respond to anti-migraine medications such as triptans do not rule out TIA or stroke.

If your spouse has symptoms of a TIA, don't wait until the morning or the next day. Strokes can be prevented if acted upon swiftly—especially an ischemic stroke.

What the spouse should expect to hear from the doctor when faced with a TIA:

- Is this a TIA or a migraine headache?
- Did the patient have a brain hemorrhage or is the TIA caused by ischemic event due to blockage of the arteries in the brain? (85 percent of TIA and strokes are ischemic.)
- What tests should be performed in the emergency room?

The latest test is a spiral CAT scan obtained in several minutes. This test may not be available in all hospitals. A CAT scan can rule out bleeding into the brain. New magnetic resonance imaging (MRI) can delineate if the brain was damaged.

An ultrasound of the carotid arteries should be done to determine if these arteries on both sides of the neck that supply blood to the brain are blocked. Surgery performed on the partially blocked carotid arteries can prevent a stroke.

If there is no evidence of a hemorrhage in the brain, some medical centers are using clot busters (tissue plasminogen activator, or tPA) if the stroke is less than three hours in duration. This becomes a major decision that needs to be made with expert advice, as the tPA can convert a simple stroke to a massive brain hemorrhage.

If an embolism (or clot) traveling from the heart through-out the system is suspected as the cause of TIA, as found in atrial fibrillation, the patient is given Coumadin (a blood thin-ner) to prevent further embolisms.

If there is no cause found for the TIA, aspirin is the drug of choice, either alone or combined with the newer drug clopidogrel (Plavix).

BOWEL CANCER—
The number three killer of men

Jason was a very successful architect, but the main joy in his life was playing the saxophone on weekends or whenever he got the chance. At the age of 62 he read one of Joseph Campbell's books and the words "follow your bliss" nagged at his brain like a catchy tune. Jason was a big man—obese—and so was his wife. He was going to give up his architectural agency and play the horn.

He was a sitter, meaning for most of his adult life, during waking hours, he was seated whether it was in front of the TV, at his desk, or while playing the saxophone. One night, Jason saw a TV show, at dinnertime no less, that showed a guy not being able to sit through a concert because of his rectal itch from hemorrhoids. Jason had just that problem—itching hemorrhoids that occasionally bled. He just bought the stuff advertised on TV and felt some relief, but there was still some blood in the toilet bowl. One drop of blood in the bowl can make it look like a massive hemorrhage. Now Martha, his wife of forty years, urged him to see a doctor when she saw the blood. She checked the toilet bowl each day after Jason turned 62. She also checked the color of the sclera of his eyes, the tone of his skin, and the color of his stool and urine.

"My hemorrhoids have been bothering me," Jason told his wife, "and sometimes they bleed. If I go see a doctor he will put his finger up there and make them bleed and make it worse."

Martha read in *The New York Times* that in a study conducted at the University of Chicago only a minority of men take advantage of the prevention testing for cancer of the intestine; Jason wasn't one of these men. He had his own ideas about health and would not listen to his wife. He bought some witch hazel in Essex, Connecticut, and applied it to his hemorrhoids the same way his father used to do to treat his "purple devils." It worked: the bleeding, itching, and pain stopped. Martha still insisted he see "the rear admiral"—a doctor who specializes on that part of the body and hemorrhoids.

Unfortunately, Jason did not get to see a doctor until he had a massive hemorrhage from his rectum one night. A large cancer was found easily within reach of the doctor's examining finger. By then the cancer had spread to his liver, but with excellent treatment, he lived a few more years. Unfortunately, the cancer caught up with him and he died in the prime of his life.

If found early, cancer of the colon is a curable disease. Here is what the spouse can do for herself and her husband to detect an early cancer. (Note: Cancer of the colon is even more common in women.)

Testing for blood in the stool during a self-hemacult rectal examination is the cheapest and least accurate. It can detect cancer 33 percent of the time, according to the Harvard Center for Cancer Prevention.

How is the test performed? The subject must use hemacult cards and smear feces on a card each day for three days and then send them to a laboratory for analysis.

Aspirin and other anti-inflammatory agents such as ibuprofen can cause slight bleeding and make the test positive. Patients are advised not to take these products several days before performing the fecal blood test. Also, Vitamin C in dosages greater than 250 mg can mask the presence of blood in the stools.

Forty-five percent of cancer of the bowel begins at the lower third of the bowel, which can be discovered by a simple scope passed through the rectum, called a flexible sigmoid-scope.

The colonoscopy is the most thorough examination of the bowel as this flexible tube examines the entire length of the colon. A barium X-ray can also visualize the entire bowel. The sad news is that some HMOs and Medicare do not reimburse preventive colonoscopy to save your life. They scream to the public that the road to preventive medicine must be practiced, yet they will not pay for real preventive measures such as a colonoscopy or a routine exercise stress test to detect narrowed coronary arteries.

The guidelines that warrant a full colon exam are:

- rectal bleeding or blood found in the stool;
- cramps or lasting abdominal pain;
- change in bowel habits that last four or five days (e.g., diarrhea, constipation, or narrowing of stool).

The American Cancer Society recommends the following for detection of rectocolon cancer for men and women over the age of 50:

- Yearly blood stool test.
- Sigmoidoscopy every five years.
- Colonoscopy every ten years.

High-risk individuals with a strong family history of cancer of the bowel or polyps should have colonoscopy examinations before the age of 50—and repeated exams according to the advice of the doctor. If the HMO refuses to pay for a colonoscopic examination, insist on getting the refusal in writing so that if an advanced cancer shows up, you have a record of the refusal.

Will diet prevent cancer of the bowel? For years we were all encouraged to eat high-bulk grains. Now this practice is not believed to prevent cancer of the bowel.

More than 90 percent of people survive colorectal cancer if detected early. Today only 38 percent of cases are discovered early. Cancer of the bowel is a silent disease until it reaches a fatally advanced stage.

Justice Ruth Bader Ginsburg of the Supreme Court was discovered to suffer from cancer after she experienced symptoms initially misdiagnosed as diverticulitis. Her diagnosis and openness helped to give a wakeup call for Americans to get screening for cancer of the colon. The same can be said for the courage and persistence of Katie Couric, whose husband passed away prematurely from the disease.

WEAKNESS AND FATIGUE

A miraculous creation, an absolute perfect working system defines our body. Each molecule of our body serves multiple purposes. Miles and miles of tracts of vessels, nerves, muscles, and tendons are interconnected with the main power station of the brain. Our internal pharmacy with millions of chemicals may never be duplicated in spite of the genius of new gene production. We introduce the worst poisons to our beautiful, wondrous, balanced systems, such as cigarettes, drugs, and other chemicals—and then we need pharmaceutical products to try to correct the malfunctions of our disturbed organs.

Our body sends out messages to us that we often do not recognize. It cries out for help in the form of pain, fever, loss of appetite, and fatigue. New onset of continued weakness and fatigue is one of the earliest signals that something has changed the "milieu interior," (the internal environment of the body), as Claude Bernard, the brilliant French physiologist, called it one hundred years ago.

A spouse should take heed if her husband complains of being tired and feeling weak for extended periods of time.

Energetic Wally could play three sets of tennis, run a mile, and then swim for one hour and not break a sweat. Wally became rich in the packaging business. He reasoned if people have more money than ever, they are going to spend like crazy and they will need boxes to ship their goods and purchases. He formed the Wally Box Company and the rest was history. At the age of 51, Wally sold his business for hundreds of millions of dollars to devote his time to travel and recreation.

Right after he retired, he complained of feeling weak and had a hard time getting out of bed. Before his retirement, he was a screaming maniac by five in the morning, getting ready for work. His wife a thin, tall, smart, beautiful graduate of a southern Baptist college, decided her Yankee husband was suffering from depression and sent him to see Dr. R, a shrink. "Yes," the doctor told Wally, "I do think you are suffering

from depression because you sold your hundred million dollar business and now you no longer have a goal or purpose in
life." Wally saw the shrink each week, who prescribed the best
antidepressants you can buy. Wally felt better, and at a Fourth
of July celebration at the Yacht Club, and while saluting the
red, white, and blue, Wally fell to the ground before the admiral of the yacht club gave the order "At Ease."

Wally was brought by ambulance to the hospital, where he
was found to have had a massive heart attack; he could not be
resuscitated.

Whenever I see a patient who complains of feeling weak
and tired, my first instinct is to check out his heart. Fatigue
can be a warning sign that a weakened heart is not pumping
enough blood to supply sufficient oxygen to the rest of the
body.

Infections, internal bleeding, and cancer may be preceded
by weakness and fatigue. There is always a cause for feeling
weak, besides depression. When my two daughters were
young, they would complain of "feeling poorly" sometimes,
wanting to skip school, but most of the time it was a prodro-
mal symptom of an infection brewing.

I am convinced that illnesses that incubate in our bodies
send out messages weeks, sometimes months, or perhaps years
in advance of their ugly outward appearance. Cancer of the
pancreas, liver troubles, and lymphoma, along with heart disease—the number one killer—weave their poisons insidiously.
If you could recognize the signs and symptoms early enough,
perhaps a doctor could scotch their full-blown appearance.

"Miriam," a man, who was a decorator, worked at night
in the Village as a female impersonator. He had lived with
another impersonator for ten years. When Miriam consulted
me it was for having lost all his energy and being constantly

tired. He had a voice and appearance like Marlene Dietrich, whom he imitated in the cabarets in Greenwich Village.

He was concerned that his lover was having a romance with another man and perhaps his lover had the big "A" and had infected Miriam. He consulted me also because his heart was always racing like a train. A test for HIV virus was negative and his heart tests were normal. Miriam was happy; off he went, on with his career.

One year later Miriam appeared in my office looking terrible. He had gained weight, losing his previously slim appearance. His face was swollen and he spoke like a broken record—slow and deliberate, as if he had a "frog in his throat." He complained he was always cold now, even in the middle of a scorching summer in New York. He had numbness of his effeminate hands and his eyelids were swollen, hanging down like sacs.

"I lost my voice, doctor, I feel like I have a sore throat all the time. I move like a turtle, forget about dancing," he told me. "I have not had a drink in six months and I never use any drugs. I am only 45 years old and I feel like an old man."

I examined Miriam and noticed his reflexes responded in slow motion. His skin had a pasty pale appearance, and his heart, on the X-ray, looked like a large triangular urn. His blood tests showed classical findings of advanced hypothyroidism, meaning a severely underactive thyroid gland.

It took several months of carefully administrating thyroid replacement to achieve the correct level; and in nine months Miriam was back to his own self.

An underactive thyroid gland has an insidious onset and is quite common, but often diagnosed at a later stage. It has been called the great mimicker of many illnesses because the symptoms are so varied, but the most common one is a generalized fatigue and lassitude, sometimes described as "just plain lazy and careless."

Henry, a barber, had a heart murmur since the age of ten. Some doctors heard it, others didn't. As the barber reached the age of 40, the murmur became louder. Henry was proud of his hair and kept his body trim; he also was noted for his perfect teeth, and saw a dentist every four months.

Henry bowled twice per week and played handball when the weather permitted. He was happily married and had two children away in college and he worked very hard at his profession. "Twenty-five years of barbering, and I'm getting tired of it," he told me. "Once the kids finish college, I'm through. My wife and I have been working for that day for twenty years."

Henry looked tired and pale; he was found to be slightly anemic. "I feel like I have the flu," he told me. "Everything hurts, my bones and legs and back, and it isn't the flu season. Doc, I really feel tired. I just want to sleep. Getting to work is too much of an effort . . . do I have Lyme disease?"

In the office examination Henry had a normal blood pressure and temperature, and normal X-ray. It turned out Henry had gone to his dentist for some dental work two weeks earlier. All tests were normal, even the Lyme test.

A blood culture was ordered and two days later it showed the results. Henry was suffering from endocarditis. His mitral valve was infected because the dentist failed to give Henry the prophylactic penicillin that patients with heart murmur should receive one hour before getting dental work.

He was treated for six weeks with intravenous antibiotics and was cured. Henry told us later that he had been feeling "under the weather" for weeks, perhaps months.

If your spouse has a heart murmur, insist that he receive antibiotics each time he sees a dentist, lest he contract endocarditis. This illness, before penicillin was made available, was always fatal. The mortality rate of endocarditis today is still high, especially in HIV-drug users, in spite of all the antibiotics we now have available. Don't rely on the dentist, but I do believe the dentist has an obligation to ask the patient if they have a murmur and then take the appropriate steps—but don't depend on it; ask!

SHORTNESS OF BREATH

Besides having a busy medical practice five days a week, teaching, writing books, playing tennis four to five times a week, I also love to travel. One year ago or so in the middle of June, I returned from one of my many jaunts to Paris feeling wonderful. I went right back to my busy schedule of playing tennis. Two weeks later as I ran up the stairs at Yale New Haven Hospital to get to the upper floors to see patients, I felt a little more short of breath than usual. I rarely use elevators.

While playing tennis that same day I began to huff and puff and cough each time I ran for the ball. Still, being male, and a doctor, I was quite cavalier regarding feeling short of breath. I did not rush to see a doctor.

On the weekend, I was digging in my garden to plant some rose bushes and I became short of breath with each shovel load of dirt. I did not tell my fiancée or anyone, but the following morning, climbing stairs was a serious effort. Was this a heart attack? Pneumonia? The saying goes, "The doctor who treats himself is treating a fool." Finally, I relinquished my strong, macho self-image, and visited a colleague of mine at lunchtime—only because my fiancée insisted and threatened to move back to Texas.

"Would you do me a favor?" I asked the doctor in a sheepish, apologetic manner, "Do you mind listening to my lungs? I have been so damn short of breath since I returned from Paris."

The doctor, a wise, old-fashioned clinician (these are becoming as rare as hen's teeth) listened to my lungs and heart and took an ECG.

"Well I don't hear anything in your lungs, but your heart has some louder sounds. Your pulmonary heart sound is increased."

"Do I have pulmonary embolism!" I exclaimed. "It can't be, I am too active—that happens to people who are inactive after surgery."

He ordered a special new test called a spiral scan (a fast CAT scan) which disclosed I suffered a massive pulmonary embolism (massive clots in my lungs). They also discovered I had a clot in my upper left thigh, which formed as a result of sitting on the plane for eight hours, and the clot broke off and traveled to my lungs. I was hospitalized in the intensive care unit for eight days and I received blood thinner. I was lucky to survive because the death rate from pulmonary embolism is anywhere from 40 percent or better. I also was lucky I had a smart doctor who made a quick and correct diagnosis. Pulmonary embolism is the second most common cause of sudden death in the United States.

One of my colleagues, a younger man than I, returned from a trip to Ohio and complained of a cough and shortness of breath. His wife, who was a physician, diagnosed pneumonia. An X-ray of the chest disclosed infiltrate in the lung that looked like pneumonia. With antibiotics and cough medicine the good doctor did not improve, but became progressively worse. His wife insisted that he should see a lung specialist, who eventually diagnosed a pulmonary embolism. He was treated with blood thinners for one week and returned to work taking Coumadin.

Pulmonary embolism occurs 600,000 times each year and as many as 200,000 people die each year. Often it occurs as the consequence of being bedridden after surgery, or a heart attack, and after a long plane or car ride.

Rocky, who ran a garden center, was a patient of mine who was terrified of doctors. He dreaded his upcoming hip surgery. He was very vocal, in and out of the hospital, but the nurses liked him because he was a perfect gentleman. He had his wife bring candy and gifts and flowers to the nursing staff after his hip replacement. But Rocky was considered by all that knew him to be on "the nervous side." Several days after surgery, Rocky began to hyperventilate—breathing rapidly and acting anxiously. The staff gave him Valium, which calmed him down to some degree. His wife, Nina, told the doctors, "My Rocky is a nervous type, but not *so* nervous." She read on the Internet about the complications of hip surgery, raced back to the hospital and asked the doctors in the most polite manner to look for pulmonary embolism. The young intern from Pakistan agreed with Nina's diagnosis and ordered the scan. He became the hero of the day because a massive pulmonary embolism was found on Rocky's lung.

Hyperventilation is a common symptom of pulmonary embolism and too often is mistaken for anxiety reactions. His wife and the intern saved Rocky's life. Rocky arranged for the intern, his wife and five children to take a free four-day trip to Las Vegas, including five hundred dollars to spend at the Casino.

Becoming suddenly short of breath, or of a gradual onset of shortness of breath, is one of the most common complaints in a medical practice, and one of the most arduous tasks to sort out. The spouse can provide indispensable help in the diagnosis. Men are liars, as I mentioned before, and they will not admit to the simplest actual or perceived weakness.

Albert, a 49-year-old builder of fine houses, consulted me because of shortness of breath. Luckily his wife, Kelly, came along for the interview. I asked Albert, "Do you smoke?" He answered, "Just a few once in a while." But his spouse, Kelly, said, "My husband is not telling you the truth, he smokes all day and has been coughing, and now he has trouble breathing." I looked up toward Albert, who sat in front of me like a little schoolboy in trouble, eyes toward the floor, coughing.

"How long have you been short of breath, Albert?" I was afraid of the answer. "Just today I was pulling up a tree in my back yard, and I suddenly got short of breath . . . now that's all there is to it, doc." I looked toward his wife sitting beside him waiting to hear more. She said, "That is the truth, Albert is strong as a horse. I will be dead before him. He plays cards with his buddies and comes home smelling like a wood stove, but he never complains of feeling short of breath—coughing, yes, all night, but not wheezing—and now, God, does he wheeze!"

I examined his lungs and he was wheezing; his ECG was normal. Why would a man become suddenly short of breath? A chest X-ray supplied the answer. He collapsed his lung as he pulled out the tree stump. He was admitted into the hospital and a chest tube was inserted into his chest. It took four days before his lung expanded to normal size.

As soon as Albert left the hospital, I watched him pull out a pack of cigarettes and I was certain he was going to fling them into the garbage pail. Instead, he placed one into his mouth, coughed, lit it, and drove off.

Two years later, Albert came to my office again complaining of difficulty breathing. His wife came along and the same scenario was played out again, except this time Albert suffered a massive heart attack. For two years we tried to arrange for Albert to have an exercise stress test, but there was always another important building project going on. "Hey, doc, these are good times, don't you know? I ain't going to refuse a job from some big rich mother. I will get to you, don't worry. Yeah, I'm still smoking, but I'm giving it up. I promise" He never did.

Albert's heart was so badly damaged that we could not perform a bypass operation. His only hope for survival was a heart transplant. In the meantime, he was placed on a heart assist device and, by some good fortune, he was able to receive a second-hand heart from a donor.

The operation was a success. Albert survived and left the hospital with his new heart, surrounded by his happy family and concerned wife. Four months later, Albert was back on the job, supervising multimillion dollar projects; he also started smoking again—two packs of cigarettes per day. We expected Albert to return as a patient soon.

Shortness of breath can be the earliest signal of heart failure.

B.J., an attorney-at-law, complained of being short of breath while walking on the golf course. His cronies, other lawyers, diagnosed him as being too fat, with his belly hanging over so far he had trouble seeing the little golf ball. He would turn, swing, and by instinct the club found the mark—but the lawyer huffed and puffed. Back at the 9th hole clubhouse, lawyer B.J. drank a beer and lit a cigar. He started to cough and someone yelled out, "For Christ's sake, go and see your doctor." No one knew who yelled that out, but it made everyone laugh and the staunch attorney was embarrassed. He left the clubhouse and did make an appointment to see his family doctor.

"Lose weight, give up the cigars, and your breathing will improve. That belly is just too much to carry around; you will end up having a heart attack," his doctor told him.

Now the lawyer's wife, a smart cookie, asked if the doctor performed an echocardiogram (ultrasound of the heart). She insisted her husband—the tough, brutal litigator—see a cardiologist. It turned out the lawyer was so obese that it was hard to hear a heart murmur, but the expert cardiologist whose ears were as sharp as a needle detected one. The echocardiogram revealed a critically narrowed aortic valve, and that was the main cause for the shortness of breath. After the aortic valve was replaced with an artificial valve, the belly became smaller. He stopped smoking cigars, and even his golf game improved dramatically.

SMOKING

Cigarettes kill more Americans each year than the total number of Americans killed in World War II, the Korean conflict, the Vietnam War, and the Gulf War combined. The high price of a pack of cigarettes does not seem to deter the number of smokers. The billions of dollars in settlements against the cigarette manufacturers still does not deter men and women from smoking. Smoking is the major cause of heart attacks stroke, cancer of the lung, and vascular disease. Secondary smoke probably is as dangerous to a bystander as to the person who smokes.

If your spouse still smokes, it will take a major medical near-disaster to make him give it up. Albert, the builder, did return to the hospital with his new heart and all his arteries clogged; he died suddenly. Smoking accelerates arteriosclerosis by twenty-fold, especially after a heart transplant.

Nicotine, a powerful poison, is the most addictive component of cigarette smoke. There are other poisons in cigarette smoke, such as nitrogen oxides, carbon monoxide, ammonia, nitroamines, and aromatic amines.

The two most dangerous hazards to the body are smoking and eating too much, and they are the most difficult habits to convince patients to give up. Interestingly it is not related to basic intelligence or understanding of the dangers, it is an addiction that not only hurts the smoker but also the persons nearby, often loved ones.

Once the person has given up tobacco, after years of smoking, the damage already done to the body may persist and continue. Cancer of the lung can surface and hardening of the arteries may already have occurred.

The smoker or former smoker should not rely on a plain chest X-ray to find early cancer of the lung, which can be curable. It is a difficult task to convince an HMO or Medicare to allow a routine chest X-ray, as well as a CAT scan, for early detection of cancer, even though it could possibly save a life. I know, because recently I fought a long battle with an HMO to obtain a CAT scan for a patient who turned out to have a small cancer in his lung. The patient had no symptoms, but he was a heavy smoker, and they refused to pay for the CAT scan until the cancer was found.

LEG PAIN

Leg pain is another symptom that can signal an impending disaster. Mike, who works in one of those mammoth-size discount stores that carries everything, came to see me one day. "Smiling Mike" is what his fellow workers call him because he is so happy at his job, working with building materials and helping customers with their home improvement projects. Mike is also smiling because he gave up smoking two years ago when his grandchild was born and his wife would not permit Mike to go near the baby as long as he smoked. "It's disgusting," she said, "I had to bear your stink but I won't allow my grandchild to be poisoned."

Smiling Mike used to race hundreds of yards from one end of the warehouse to the other, but one day he started to get cramps in both of his legs. At first they were mild, but as time went on it became worse and Mike had to stop and rest until the pain left his calves. He went to a chiropractor who diagnosed a sprained back, arthritis, and pressure on the nerves. Manipulations and massage made Mike feel better, but once he started trekking across the hard cement floor, the pain returned in both of his calves.

"Perhaps I should quit this job. I'm almost 62, I can get early retirement and social security. We have some savings and our house is paid for. We should enjoy life, play golf, see the grandchild more often, and even take a trip to Europe," he told his wife.

He quit his job and with a special travel package they went to Paris for the first time. They were on Champs-Élysées walking toward the Arc de Triomphe. "Just as so many great leaders have done in the past," Mike told his wife as they marched arm-in-arm like two wide-eyed, young lovers. But poor Mike could hardly walk because of the severe pain in his legs. He stopped to rest right in front of the famous Foucault Cafe and ordered a soft drink. To make matters worse, he could not get an erection in the most romantic setting of the hotel Meurice, where the great and famous once stayed.

The doctor who examined Mike in his hometown could not find pulses in his legs and with doppler examinations he concluded Mike had blockages in both limbs. The doctor also knew Mike had a 30 to 40 percent chance of having blocked arteries that supply the heart—the coronary arteries—and that was also the reason he lost his ability to get an erection.

A successful angioplasty operation was performed on the arteries of Mike's legs, and the clogged arteries of his heart. Three months later Mike could walk miles without pain and a heart attack was averted. They returned to Paris and this time he could walk the entire Champs Élysées, and make love in Paris the way it was meant to be.

Pain in the calf while walking is called intermittent claudi-cation; it means that arteries are blocked in the legs and there is a good chance that the arteries of the heart are blocked as well. This can occur years after smoking cessation and the spouse should be aware that leg pains occurring while walking or dancing can be caused by poor circulation of the arteries in the legs. It is a message sent out by the body to get help. The man must see a doctor who will perform the necessary tests to discover blockage. Sometimes the blockage can be so critical that gangrene can set in and amputation of the leg is the only hope for survival. Men who suffer from diabetes and smoke tobacco are at constant risk of arterial blockage in any part of the body.

Chapter Seven

Impotence

IMPOTENCE, the inability of the male to initiate and/or sustain an erection, is also designated as erectile dysfunction (E.D.). Until recently, E.D. was a silent epidemic that dated all the way back to Adam's arrival in the Garden of Eden.

But now we can actually treat this humiliating, degrading, and embarrassing male disability. Today it is no longer silent; it screams at us nightly on television. Ethical family man Senator Bob Dole has told us on national TV that he became impotent after his prostate surgery, but Viagra solved his problem.

Dozens of clinics run by lay people in the United States sprang up for the treatment of E.D. One in particular comes to mind: in rural Clanton, Alabama, there is the Norfolk Men's Clinic, owned by Anita Yates, and the clinic sells the little blue pills to help impotent men all over the world as far as Australia and Eastern Europe. This same county is best known for growing peaches and selling them on country stands—until 1998, of course, when it gained a sexy reputation.

Woe to the man in this day and age who is impotent. I suspect many relationships and marriages have been torn apart because the male was impotent and, before Viagra, most patients did not know there were other treatments available for E.D. I have heard many a wife tell me, "He did not fulfill his marital duties."

Impotence is a symptom and not a disease. However, a disease can cause impotence. In the case of Senator Dole and others like him, prostate surgery made him impotent.

Before your spouse jumps on the bandwagon of this new miracle drug, he must first be sure that he is carefully examined by a doctor who will look for a cause and not be too ready with his prescription pad. Some doctors seem to turn to the new magic drug before all the questions are answered. "I know, I know, my good man. I understand; say no more. I will fix everything; trust me."

Now take the story of Tony, who was a stud par excellence. His reputation preceded him, so to speak. Not only was he a rough looking macho man, but, in the circle of those in the know, it was reported that he had a very long sexual organ—so long, in fact, that it was legendary. The eyes of young maidens roamed over his body to the legendary spot and were envious of the lucky women who were so satisfied. Tony felt a certain strength and potency from being born the night of the two full moons.

But disaster struck one glorious June night, when Tony was about to make another conquest of a magnificent maiden from the village of X. Poor Tony's scepter of love became like a wet Chinese noodle instead of the usual staghorn. Word got around fast and Tony became morose. "As goes my scepter of love, so goes all my power," he lamented.

Historically, and to the present day, impotence erroneously is identified with loss of masculinity and strength. In biblical times, a king's power was directly linked to fertility and potency. Tony knew his bible and read in the Old Testament that when fair young virgins did not restore King David's erection, he stepped down from the throne in favor of virile Adonijah.

Surely, Tony cried out to the moon, someone had the evil eye on him. He went to see many of the elders, and finally sought the advice of an excellent internist, educated far up north. A traditional doctor-with his eyes as sharp as an eagle, his heart as strong as a lion, his hands as gentle as a dove, and his brain as fast as the newest computers—discovered that Tony had a large aneurysm growing in his belly. The aorta in the abdomen was large as a floating balloon at a fair, and it cut off the supply of blood to his large penis. Straight away, Tony was operated on, the aneurysm was removed before it burst, and Tony returned to his village, and the legend lives on and on and on.

The message here is that E.D. (erectile dysfunction) can be a sign of an impending vascular disaster such as an abdominal aneurysm or a severe peripheral vascular insufficiency, as seen in smokers and persons with high blood pressure.

Kelly, a big shot lawyer, went to see his family doctor with the complaint, "I am just not myself anymore. I am tired, I lost all my energy." The good experienced doctor cut through all that and asked one question: "Kelly, let's get to the real problem. You have trouble getting an erection, right, and you want a hormone shot."

"You got that right, Doc," Kelly said. But the wise doctor spent a good hour going over Kelly, and discovered that Kelly was on the "sauce" too much. "But only on weekends, your honor, er . . . I mean, doctor." Kelly was not convinced that alcohol, even in small amounts, can cause the penis to become limp when it should be hard.

The wise doctor, a scholar no less, quoted Shakespeare to Kelly. The quote came from Macbeth, Act II, scene 3:

MacDuff: What three things does drink especially provoke?
Porter: Merry, sir, nose-painting, and urine. Lechery, sir, it provokes, and unprovokes; it provokes the desire, but it takes away the performance.

"What that means, Kelly," the doctor translated for him, "is that even Shakespeare knew that too much booze and your penis loses."

Kelly stopped drinking because his wife threatened to leave him. His sexual abilities returned enough to satisfy his wife, who also was called Kelly. The sex life of Kelly, the lawyer, was returned to what it ince was.

Another patient of mine, KK, was a hard-working investment advisor. He had the same look on his face as that on a hundred-dollar bill. When he spoke of money he actually drooled, especially when it came to treasury bills, notes, and foreign exchange. Sooner or later he would develop hypertension; he did, and received the best drugs for hypertension. Being a tight-lipped Yankee he was too embarrassed to tell anyone that his pencil-shaped penis could not be aroused, even by the strippers in the clubs of New York.

"Dear, why not tell Paul, your doctor? Perhaps he can help you—after all dear, I am still young—58 is not old today," his wife begged him. It took three years, one divorce, a new woman, and a new doctor to convince him to get a check up. This time, his doctor did some tests. He swiftly diagnosed Kelly's problem; the beta-blockers and the diuretics he was taking for his blood pressure caused it. Several weeks later—and a romantic trip to Martha's Vineyard—his power returned.

K.K. was not ashamed to tell his problem to his new doctor whom he did not know, but was embarrassed to discuss his sexual failure with his previous family doctor who was also his friend for years and even a friend of someone important on Cape Cod.

Medications, especially tranquilizers, anti depressants, and those we use to treat hypertension or heart failure, often cause impotence.

L.B.'s wife finally left him because he abused her verbally for years. He was a miserable, egotistical guy who embarrassed his wife on all social occasions. Once he became upset with her because she did not serve the wine to their guest first. "Haven't you learned yet that guests get served first?" he said right in front of everyone. She smiled quietly—and at that moment she made her plans to leave him.

L.B., from then on, went from one affair to another, because he was rich and not bad looking, but money could not straighten out his limp penis and the young women would not tolerate his failure to make love the "old fashioned way." He finally consulted a sex therapist advertised in one of those throwaway papers. "Surrogate sex therapist . . . in the large city . . . on the third floor of an old brownstone . . . complete discretion." The therapist was trying to initiate sex with L.B., but it failed. She was optimistic for several more sessions at two-hundred-fifty-dollars a half-hour: "It will happen." That experience only added to L.B.'s increasing despair. He confided to an old Harvard classmate, now a famous politician, who told him about a legitimate psychiatrist who was an expert on sex. It turned out L.B. was suffering from depression because of his divorce and bad marriage, mostly caused by himself because "he acted like a jerk." After several months of "coming clean" about his selfish life, he improved. His depression lifted and when the next relationship appeared at his doorstep, L.B. became a marvelous lover and lived happily ever after.

Depression is a common cause of erectile dysfunction and can parade in men as fatigue, muscle pain, back pain, memory loss, and loss of interest in football, basketball, and baseball—now that is a serious symptom for us Americans.

In the United States at least 30 million American men have some degree of erectile impairment, and the number is increasing because more and more men are owning up to this illness. The Massachusetts Male Aging Study (MMAS) revealed that 52 percent of men between the ages of 40 and 70 have some form of E.D. As the man ages, E.D. increases. Now the term E.D. includes not only the inability to initiate an erection or sustain one, but also loss of sexual desire, premature ejaculation, and no ejaculation at all.

The physiology of the male penis going from flaccid to hard is very complex and as we learn more and more about it we wonder about the miracle that it hardens in the first place. It is useful for the spouse to understand that much goes into making her guy erect.

The major vessel columns surrounding the penis consist of small and large arteries, and veins are constricted when the penis is flaccid. Erection begins when the erectile center in the brain is activated and neural signals are transmitted through the spinal cord to a neuromuscular package located in the corpus cavernosum (the bulk of the penis) that houses the blood vessels. The chemical nitric oxide is released, which relaxes the blood vessels in the penis and increases the blood flow in the arteries of the penis, and at the same time shuts down the escape of blood through the veins in the penis, causing the erection. In other words, this causes blood to come to the penis and be trapped in the penis forcing the erection to take place.

It can then be understood that anything that interferes with the function of the arteries or veins of the penis, such as arteriosclerosis, excess alcohol, drugs administered for hypertension, diabetes, decreased male hormones, and, above all, smoking, can prevent an erection.

Currently, it is found that most older men with E.D. have an underlying organic cause. Previously, it was thought E.D. had mostly a psychological cause. How wrong we doctors were.

Once E.D. is improved or cured, the quality of life rises dramatically. Anger, frustration, and impatience decrease; concentration and joy of living increase.

So how can you help manage this problem if your man lost his erection? There is a natural tendency for all of us, if our sexual life dies, to blame one another. "He (or she) no longer loves me," or, "I no longer attract him," or, "He has a girlfriend"—on and on goes this litany of excuses. If the man still loves his wife and does not have a weekly rendezvous with someone else, or has found a new sexual identity (i.e., he really is gay), and does not get an erection upon mechanical stimulation (oral or masturbation), the wife must gently recommend to her spouse that he see a solidly interested family doctor who will initiate all the testing necessary to rule out a medical cause.

The important question the doctor will ask is whether or not the man gets a spontaneous morning erection. If so, it implies the mechanics of an erection are intact, but something is inhibiting the erection when it is needed. The doctor should perform a thorough physical examination and order certain basic tests; for example:

1. Endocrine cause: get thyroid functions, test for diabetes and testosterone levels.
2. Vascular cause: check the circulation of the legs and heart.
3. Alcohol and smoking evaluation.
4. Mental state: Is there depression?
5. Refer him to a urologist to check the prostate and the penis.
6. Drugs associated with impotence (already mentioned), including lipid-lowering agents, non-steroidal anti-inflammatory agents such as ibufuren, and H2 receptor blockers such as Tagamet, Prilosec, etc.
7. An open conversation with the wife and husband is helpful to see if there are some marriage problems that have not come to light. If there is a lot of anger in the marriage it will be difficult to become passionate at night if the anger begins at breakfast. As one woman psychiatrist remarked so succinctly, "Love making begins in the morning." If anger and yelling starts in the morning at the breakfast table it may very well carry through all day, and then sexual desire is blunted and no erection may be possible.

As mentioned earlier in the text, aging is a poor excuse for not being able to get an erection, unless the nefarious arteriosclerosis has set in—even then doctors can help.

How to treat impotence:

After a thorough diagnostic evaluation your mate should move right on to the first line of treatment, which is sildenafil, known to all as Viagara, the miracle drug for men. Years ago I told some of my suffering male patients, "Be patient; soon a drug company will find the magic pill that scientists have been searching for since biblical times." Every imaginable concoction has been tried to treat erectile dysfunction. In Korea, American men were given homogenized bull testicles by their girlfriends, sperm oil, male hormone injections, B12, zinc, procaine shots, hypnotism, psychotherapy. The list is endless, and all of no avail except for the placebo effect that occasionally occurs.

My father said that when his doctor gave him the testosterone injections it invigorated his sex life and he insisted that his doctor give the oral testosterone pill to give him "strength." Then he tried Vitamin E and that worked for him also. Were he alive now he would have been in paradise with the new drug.

The effectiveness of Viagra varies between 43 percent and 89 percent. Diabetic men have less of a response. Seven out of every ten doses administered yielded an erection strong enough to make penetration possible.

I inform the spouses that Viagra does not increase the sexual desire but gives the guy the confidence to move ahead, instead of turning his back on you and saying, "I'm too tired." Ideally the drug is given either at a 100 or 50 mg dosage. I usually prescribe 100 mg and instruct the man to take the full dosage and if success follows, then I ask him to try 50 mg dosage (half of the 100 mg).

In some cases it should be taken one hour before starting sex, though sometimes a longer time is needed. Alcohol is to be avoided the night of sex. Sometimes the older male finds that if he takes 50 mg of Viagra several hours earlier and then repeats the dosage five hours or so later, then his early morning erection is much stronger. After all, we men have had our early morning erections since childhood, due in part because of full bladders and because our testosterone level is the highest in the morning. Some women and men, too. do not care for the morning lovemaking and rely on the night, when fatigue and/or alcohol reign, and erection is difficult.

Patients should not take Viagra if they are also taking nitro-glycerine tablets or patches. Shortly after a heart attack or bypass operation Viagra should be withheld from patients with low blood pressure, aortic valve disease, or heart failure. If taken after a large fatty meal, its onset would be delayed. Your own doctor should be consulted before you try this drug.

The side effects are not serious; when they do occur, they consist of flushing of the face (red face), headaches, seeing blue if you look outside. Death from using Viagra has no greater incidence than a placebo.

Other oral agents recently approved are called apomor-phines. In up to 6 percent of patients it caused vomiting and in 17 percent it caused nausea. Now that would shut down any sexual desire for the spouse or the guy. Imagine, just when you are about to start a blissful night of romance, the male vomits all over you while his penis finally rises up.

If oral medication fails, there are other alternatives that the spouse should know about. There is a vacuum pump that looks like a large test tube inserted over the penis, and the pump is used to push the blood into the penis.

The FDA has approved alprostadil or prostaglandin, a vasodilator agent either injected directly into the shaft of the penis or directly into the urethral opening (the exit spot of urine and sperm). It works and is well tolerated but not to be used more than three times per week. The erection begins usually within ten minutes and lasts up to one hour. The urol-ogist will teach your mate how to give the injection and observe your lover in this task. If possible, the spouse should be present to give a helping hand if needed.

We can look forward in the future for more effective medications and safer ones to help the male maintain an active sexual life as he becomes older.

Perhaps we will no longer hear the common statements, "I am too old for sex," "I'm not interested," or "My wife and I haven't had sex for years."

Chapter Eight

The Number One Killer of Men

"DO YOU HAVE TO PLAY TENNIS TODAY?" his wife asked her husband as he was stuffing his tennis bag with his sneakers, white socks, underwear, white tennis shorts and shirt. "It is going to be hot and the humidity is over 80 percent; remember, you are 62 years old."

"Stop worrying so much," said Big Jim, "I am in great shape. I have my Saturday morning game with Ed, and I am not going to cancel because of a little humidity."

Big Jim's father died of a heart attack at the age of 62 on such a hot humid day in July, as he was walking from his house to the subway station in Queens.

"I just had my physical last week," Big Jim shouted as he left the house. "I'm late, good-bye darling, I love you. See you in a few hours." It was true Big Jim did have a physical with his private doctor, but his HMO would not approve a cardiac stress test because Big Jim was "in good shape."

Once outside of the door he began to sweat because the humidity was brutal. As he drove off in his new luxury car he cooled down with the air conditioner blowing on his body. The traffic was heavy even on this Saturday morning;

Big Jim arrived ten minutes late for his match on the court. This was a very busy tennis club; dress whites were mandatory at this old conservative club. His tall, thin partner was stretching, bending, and jumping in place, like a skeleton on Halloween.

"Let's go, Bo," Jim yelled across the court, "No warm-up! Today is your end—this is for all the marbles."

Big Jim did not bother to drink any water, and started to play his usual aggressive game. The sweat was pouring down his new tennis shirt. At the end of the first set he felt light-headed, drank some water, smiled and proceeded to attack the net with a vengeance—then, suddenly, he stopped short in his tracks and fell to the ground.

"Heat stroke," somebody yelled. The tennis pro carried some ice water to the man lying down on the ground, but Big Jim had already died of a cardiac arrest. An autopsy was performed and disclosed that all the arteries to his heart were blocked.

Could Big Jim's death have been avoided?

Lester, a well-known malpractice lawyer, had funny feelings in his chest for several weeks, during a court trial and when he jogged for ten minutes in the morning. He decided to consult his internist but never told him he was having chest discomfort.

"Let's see how bright this guy is," he said to himself. "If I tell him I'm getting chest pains, before you know it I will get a cardiac catheterization."

The doctor had the lawyer fill out a form and then the doctor asked if he had chest pain. "Not yet," the lawyer responded. His doctor believed men of fifty years and older should have a screening exercise stress test every few years or so. The lawyer agreed to undergo a stress test, but he did not tell the doctor he was having chest pain at the onset of the test. He wanted to see "what it would show." As his heart rate increased, his blood pressure suddenly fell and the lawyer collapsed on the treadmill.

"I should have told you I was having chest pains," he whispered. "I wanted to see if the machine would pick it up." The stress laboratory was prepared for heart arrests—but all the efforts of resuscitation failed.

Could this lawyer's life have been saved?

Doctor R, a wonderful cardiologist and an excellent diagnostician, was trained at one of the best medical schools, but he did not believe that a low-cholesterol and low-fat diet mattered. His wife respected him, loved him, but she regarded her husband as a "pompous ass." She believed all the statistics; she and her family followed a low-fat diet. But not "Rudolph the Doctor," the cardiologist from Vienna, who insisted that bratwurst, pig's feet, ham, salami, bacon, and eggs were a part of his heritage and should be in his daily diet. He was against smoking, but believed that drinking German ale was good for the soul and perhaps the heart—or so he proselytized.

A random sample of his cholesterol at the annual heart meeting in Dallas, Texas, showed Rudolph had very high cholesterol. "Are you now convinced, Herr Professor? Will you go on a low-fat diet?"

"Yes, my love, anything to make you happy," he told her. The good doctor never exercised except once a week on Sunday. He took a little walk on Sunday in the park, walking arm in arm with his charming wife, Hilda.

In spite of his wife's efforts, Doctor Rudolph developed angina, refused a stress test, and one fine afternoon I was called to see Rudolph because he was having a heart attack; he died in his office.

Could the cardiologist's life have been saved today?

Willard, happy Willard, loved the road, driving in his huge four-wheeler. With his window closed, he smoked in the cab of his truck, stopped at all the "greasy spoons" for ham and eggs in the morning, double hamburger with fries for lunch and, on the road, a good two-pound steak with mashed potatoes for dinner. Willard did not use the back of his truck for a bedroom to entertain the ladies of the night, but for sleep. He loved his wife and children and planned to retire to Orlando when he reached the age of 58.

Willard passed his required truck driver's test given by the doctor appointed for truckers. His blood pressure was 165 systolic and he was thirty pounds overweight, "but strong as a horse" he told the doctor. "I always get nervous during my physical; don't let that blood pressure scare you," he insisted.

"If only he had kept the appointment that I made with his regular family doctor. If only I insisted on going with him that Thursday," his wife lamented at the funeral—because Willard died shortly after his physical. He drove his truck down an embankment and the autopsy disclosed that the main artery (left main) to his heart was clogged.

Could Willard's life have been saved?

Stucci, the runner and ballplayer, even at the age of fifty, still played basketball "one on one," and baseball with the boys twenty years his junior. Stucci always had an ugly, smelly, black cigar dangling from his mouth. His body, his car, his clothing stank from the tobacco. His wife, Dora, hated the smell and forced him to smoke on the porch that he had built ten years earlier. He was not allowed to smoke near his grandchildren and Dora made him bathe, scrub his body with a special violet soap, followed with jasmine, before he held his precious grandchildren in his arms.

"Enough is enough," so he told Dora, "I will quit smoking at Lent." He did. She cheered, the grandchildren danced around and around him. Stucci (short for Smelly) quit and got his old name back: Leonardo.

Money was saved from not smoking, and they lived happily until one morning at the gym. Leonardo felt pain in his calf after running for a ball. When he stopped short, the pain stopped. The pain, not present at rest, surfaced each time he walked.

"Arthritis finally got me," he told his wife. She "dragged" him to the doctor not only because of his "arthritis," but because Leonardo's penis was limp like a noodle. This was not discussed with the doctor.

The doctor said that Leonardo had poor circulation in his legs and told him that it was due to more than thirty-five years of smoking. He was treated for the poor circulation of his legs, which improved, but poor Leonardo cried in the emergency room as he was being treated for a massive heart attack one year later.

"I gave up smoking to avoid a heart attack and look what happened!" But he was lucky; his life was saved by the excellent, miraculous treatment of today. Alas, giving up smoking after years and years of this disgusting habit leaves behind the after-effects of injured lungs and arteries all over the body, as we have seen in the story of Leonardo.

All is not lost. Stop smoking today and the cells will become clean and fresh if you stop early enough. If not, we can still repair things as we did with Leonardo.

IN THE PRECEDING STORIES, some of the men died suddenly without any warning. In up to 25 percent or more of sudden death cases, there are no initial symptoms of coronary artery disease! Interestingly, more than 60 percent had consulted a physician because of unrelated problems.

In hospitals that do not have a chest pain center, up to 20 percent of patients are sent home with the missed diagnosis of a heart attack. Even more startling is that one-third of acute myocardial infarction patients are present without chest pain.

Right at this point, I urge the spouse to challenge the emergency room doctor or family doctor to be certain her man is not having a heart attack. *Say*, "Are you sure he is not having a heart attack?" *Say it*, even if your man does not have chest pain, but his only complaint is shortness of breath. I will discuss this in detail following.

There are at least six million people who visit emergency rooms for chest pain each year. Heart attacks are diagnosed in about 15 percent of patients. However, to make things even more difficult for the doctor, an estimated 40 percent of patients who come in with chest pain turn out not to have a heart attack.

Today, 1.5 million people experience a heart attack each year and 500,000 die! The good news is that in the past twenty-five years there has been an age-adjusted decrease by 45 percent of deaths from a heart attack.

Now, time out for a few definitions that even we doctors need to review:

What is a heart attack (myocardial infarction) anyway?

When the arteries to the heart (the coronary arteries) are critically blocked, and no blood flows through carrying the oxygen needed by the heart muscle, the muscle is damaged or dies. This is called a heart attack. The classical symptoms are chest pain, profuse sweating accompanied by shortness of breath, and a feeling of impending doom. At the time, the victim may collapse or have minimal symptoms or none at all. The muscle of the heart may become entirely destroyed unless some swift treatment is given, or if the injury is only slight.

What is heart failure?

The heart, once called "the seat of the soul" (so named by Aristotle), is a muscle. This precious muscle governs life. It can become weakened by a heart attack, or destroyed by viruses or by leaking heart valves. The heart may also become thinned out, dilated, or thickened by long-standing hypertension—called hypertrophy.

If its pumping action fails, then the blood that is returned back to the heart remains imprisoned in the heart chambers. It has to go somewhere, so the heart compensates by enlarging—this is called cardiomegaly. The blood backs up into the lungs and the person complains of shortness of breath and fatigue. This is what is meant by heart failure.

We can measure the degree of heart muscle damage by various techniques such as echocardiography or a nuclear scan. We can then derive a functional unit of the heart muscle called the ejection fraction. If this number is low, such as 25 percent, it means the heart is severely damaged, and this results in heart failure. The ejection fraction gives doctors guidelines to select the best treatment.

Heart failure is one of the leading causes of death today. It is a challenge for the cardiologist to try to extend the patient's life using all the modern medications now available. Once heart failure has set in the death rate can be close to 40 percent. Now with new medications, we have improved our success rate and prolonged patients' lives considerably.

Sometimes a heart transplant can be the only alternative for the patient if all treatment fails, providing numerous criteria are present. Age is one of the many critical factors that determine whether a patient receives a transplant, or not.

What is a coronary thrombosis or a coronary?

This term has the same meaning as a heart attack.

What is angina or an angina attack?

If the coronary arteries (arteries that supply the heart) become blocked or go into spasm, a classical type of chest pain occurs called angina attack. It is a warning sign that a catastrophe may be in the making.

Angina pectorals, translated from the Latin, means "pain in the chest." It is a distinctive pain, usually situated behind the breastbone, radiating out to the left side of the chest, down the inner side of the left arm, or radiating to the jaw, wrist, or back. It can be precipitated by effort, emotional strain or excitement, and relieved by rest and nitroglycerine. It is a heavy feeling in the chest, described by some men "as if someone is sitting on my chest." It can be quite severe, often accompanied by sweating. The pain may be mild and, thus, dismissed as slight indigestion, or can it be like a sensation of strangulation, choking, panic, and despair. Angina is a transient symptom in contrast to heart attack or myocardial infarction. It can occur as a result of effort or emotional strain or excitement. It can be precipitated by anxiety, cold, exercise, climbing stairs, shoveling snow, playing active sports, or having sexual activity.

What are the coronary arteries?

Galen, the anatomist, was the doctor for gladiators in the second century A.D. He used the term "coronary" to describe the arteries that supply the heart. At the end of a tournament, Galen cut the beating heart out of a dying victim and ran through the gladiator arena showing off the beating heart to the cheering Romans in the amphitheater. He was a young doctor looking for work. Little did he know he set the stage for open heart surgery hundreds of years later.

Leonardo da Vinci, in the year 1452, sketched the artery vessels in the way we are accustomed to seeing them today.

Notions of the coronary arteries go back even further to ancient Egypt, where they were described to some degree in papyrus scrolls.

What is an arrhythmia?

Skipped beats, missed beats, palpitations, or extra systole beats, all mean the same thing, but may have different implications. An arrhythmia can also mean a rapid regular beat, or an irregular beat. Sometimes it kills the person.

What is cardiac catheterization or angiography?

This is a method of X-ray visualization of the heart and the coronary arteries, the valves, and the heart muscle.

What is the genesis of blocked arteries that leads to clots, also called thrombi, followed by a heart attack?

I will briefly outline the events to show what the spouse can do to prevent a heart attack.

Normal arteries rarely become blocked. Arteries that are diseased with arthrosclerosis are the ones that become thrombosed. Arthrosclerosis, to distinguish it from arteriosclerosis (loss of elastic tissue from the walls of the arteries), is caused by lipoproteins such as LDL being deposited in the walls of arteries. These liquid deposits of fat lead to the formation of plaque—which is not unlike the plaque on your teeth. The LDL (low-density lipoprotein, the bad cholesterol from our diet) enters the wall of the artery, becomes modified and oxidized. It results in smooth muscle growth; calcium and the platelets from the blood are attracted to this nidus, like bees to honey, and the plaque grows larger. The covering of the artery called the endothelium—once thought to be nothing but inert tissue—turns out to be an important active tissue. The integrity of the endothelium depends on nitric oxide. Normal arterial endothelial produces lots of nitric oxide, and the artery dilates or widens; those impaired by plaque formation and decreased nitric oxide production can't dilate and blood flow diminishes or even ceases. This is an over-simplification of a complex physiological and pathological happening at the arterial level.

Thrombi develop on these plaques. If the plaques are soft, they can rupture and cause an open door for the formation of clots consisting of platelets and other substances such as fibrin and LDL.

The more LDL available to the artery, the easier it will be for plaque to congregate, increasing the potential for clots or thrombi to form. The plaque becomes thrombogenic. It attracts all the bad things in our blood that mostly come from the fats we ingest. Thus, thrombosis blocks the coronary arteries and a heart attack (myocardial infarction) develops.

What possibly can prevent the clot from forming and rupturing?

We know the higher the cholesterol and the LDL, the greater danger of plaque formation. The earliest signs of arthrosclerosis, consisting of fatty streaks, have been found at age of 18 to 25 in American men.

One recent study of data from autopsies performed on young American boys, who died as results of accidents, found that 25 percent of them showed the beginning of plaque buildup in their arteries. Similar studies were conducted on American soldiers killed in Korea and Vietnam, which found the arteries streaked with fat; but none were found among killed Korean or Vietnamese men of the same age.

In all cases I cited above, preventive measures might have saved their lives. Thirty-five years ago or so, 800,000 deaths occurred yearly from heart attacks alone. Today we have dropped the yearly death rate to 450,000, but the heart attack rate remains as high as in bygone days. Perhaps it is even higher today, since we are living longer and can save most people who have sustained a heart attack if they arrive early enough at the hospital.

Here are some of the well-known preventive measures you, the wife, can get your man to practice:

Your spouse should know what level his cholesterol (LDL and HDL) is in the blood. It is not enough to buy a kit or have a doctor that just measures your cholesterol. It's like measuring just the gasoline in your car but without knowing if it needs oil.

I have asked dozens and dozens of patients, including doctors, lawyers, and other professional men and women, if they know what their cholesterol level is. Most didn't know and very few even heard of the bad cholesterol measurements called the LDL—the culprit that is responsible for plaque formation. So be sure the entire lipid profile is ordered by your doctor. This profile should include cholesterol, HDL, LDL, and triglyceride levels.

HDLs are scavengers—they mop up the LDL before it becomes oxidized and congregated in an artery. The higher the HDL level is in the blood (50 or greater) the less chance of a heart attack. The higher the LDL, the greater the risk for a heart attack.

For primary prevention I aim at a LDL below 100 and the same for secondary prevention (i.e., after a heart attack, angioplasty, or bypass surgery). Ideally, an LDL below 90 is the key to keeping plaque levels low and to prevent it from congregating. A low LDL level also helps strengthen its texture, preventing it from rupturing, and allowing a clot to form.

A good cholesterol level is below 180. Most men who have had heart attacks have cholesterol readings of 230 or so; with LDL of 170, or higher; and triglycerides of 300 or better.

Diet is the first move toward saving your spouse's life once you know the fat levels in his blood. The purpose of the diet is to lower the LDL. I recommend that total fat intake should not exceed 35 percent—10 percent saturated and no more than 10 percent unsaturated. The average American eats 800 milligrams of fat per day or more. Your husband's intake of fat should not exceed 200 mg. My diet (see Appendix) will reduce the overall blood cholesterol by 20 to 50 percent, and the LDL by 15 to 20 percent.

A recent study in Lyon, France (a city with the lowest heart attack and death rate in the Western world), found persons who eat more bread, beans, fiber, poultry, fish, and canola oil, and less meat, butter, and cream, were less susceptible to cardiac deaths by 65 percent.

Most of the saturated fats in meat are palmitic, which raises the LDL cholesterol. In dairy foods, myristic saturated fat raises the LDL even more than the palmitic.

The good fats are the nonsaturated fats, such as those found in olive oil and walnuts; they tend to lower the LDL and the cholesterol.

Polyunsaturated fatty acids, such as those found in corn, soybean, safflower oils, and fish, lower the LDL level.

The fat story is confusing to the reader as well as to us doctors; all fats contain the good and the bad, and you have to choose the ones that are the best.

My diet, called the Kra Diet, which will be found in the appendix, is a perfect, well-balanced diet to prevent heart attacks and sudden death. Vegetables and fish and one glass of red wine along with lower calorie intake, are the excellent preventive guidelines.

Some studies recently have reported that walnuts, rich in nonsaturated fats, coupled with a diet of fish and vegetables, helped to reduce the LDL.

Smoking cigars, cigarettes, and pipes also adversely affect

these levels. If your spouse stops smoking, it will raise up his HDL and lower the LDL levels.

Exercise also elevates the HDL and lowers the LDL to some degree.

After all is said and done about diets, exercise and stopping smoking, the final best proven way to lower the dangerous LDL levels is with medications. There is still a very large resistance to the use of drugs to lower the fats in the blood, by the public and doctors. "I am afraid of side-effects like liver damage and other problems reported," is the rationale used by patients.

Every drug has potential side effects, usually low and rare, but the side effect of high LDL and low HDL can be early death.

Currently, the most popular and effective drugs used to lower fatty poisons in our blood are called the HMG-CoA reductase inhibitors referred to as statins—lovastatin was the first, followed by pravastatin, simvastin, fluvastatin, atorvastatin, and cerivastatin. All these statins reduce the incidence of heart attacks or, to put it another way, delay the onset of heart attacks. They decrease the synthesis in the liver of cholesterol, accelerate LDL reduction and removal from the blood circulation system, and improve the endothelial function, as discussed above.

The major side effect in my experience has been joint and muscle pains. These symptoms subside as soon as the medication is discontinued. When I had my lipid profile tested years ago, I had a LDL of 170, and cholesterol of 220. My family doctor started me on one of the statins and I was jumping with joy because six weeks later my LDL dropped to 90, the cholesterol dropped to 170, and my HDL skyrocketed to 50.

One year later, I began to have aches in my back and legs after a single tennis match. "What do you expect," a colleague said, "as we get older the joints and muscles go." For one week I played no tennis and sat around watching sports on television. I became downhearted and missed my tennis matches. My back and legs ached more than before.

My sweet wife urged me to see a bone specialist, who told me, "You have early arthritis, old chap. Ease up on tennis, play doubles." I did as I was told and it just happened that I ran out of the statins I was taking and it took one week before my prescription was refilled. Well, lo and behold, all my muscle pains subsided and, sure enough, the statins were responsible for the pains.

Then I tried niacin, a vitamin medication that has been around for fifty years. I often prescribe it to my patients if their cholesterol is too high and the triglycerides are out of sync. It raises the HDL, and lowers the LDL. I know not to use it with diabetics because it increases the insulin requirements and it is not to be used by patients who have liver problems.

I bought the vitamin over the counter on one hot summer day and I took a 500 mg dosage. I climbed into my car and about fifteen minutes later my body became hot and my face red as a lobster. When I got home I tore off my clothing and, as my wife and children watched curiously, I dove into our pool to cool off.

Niacin, I remembered, can cause an intolerable temperature increase and redness of the body, as happened to me. Niacin was discovered by Dr. Goldberger who used it to treat pellagra, which is a nutritional ailment resulting from poor food intake. Alas, as safe and effective as niacin is, I could not tolerate it.

Fish oil tablets are not recommended unless the triglycerides are high. Diabetics need to be especially careful as it can increase the tendency to bleed.

I munched on walnuts and tried the statins again, but at a lower dosage and only three times a week. I got the same excellent results of lowering my LDL with no muscle or joint pains (except on occasions when I play a long single match and lose).

Clofibrate, another agent used for high triglycerides, may cause cancer of the GI tract. Likewise, the one-time darling of the lipid-lowering drugs, fibric acid derivatives, cause too many side effects to be used, except in selected patients resistant to the statins, or in combination with statins.

It is possible that some day we will say the same thing regarding statins. For now, in the year 2001, it is the drug of choice to lower the LDL and cholesterol.

Are there other tests that should be done besides testing for lipoproteins in the blood?

There is renewed interest in the level of homocysteine in the blood. Some researchers think that elevated levels of this by-product of metabolism is more important than the cholesterol level. They claim excessive homocysteine is the real culprit that causes heart attacks, strokes, birth defects, and miscarriages. Elevated levels of homocysteine are linked to phlebitis, pulmonary embolism, and peripheral vascular disease.

The spouse should tell her husband or the doctor that while blood is drawn for lipids, a homocysteine level should be done. The normal level should be below 12; higher levels are associated with heart attacks.

Fifteen thousand doctors participated in the five-year-long Physicians Health Study. Those with a homocysteine level of 15 micromoles or higher had three times the incidence of heart attacks than those with lower levels.

The theory says that homocysteine, an amino acid, damages the artery and, thus, cholesterol plaques can readily form.

You can lower your spouse's homocysteine level by urging him to eat less meat and to take daily folic acid B6 and B12, even if his homocysteine level is below 12. A recent study suggested 5 mg of folic acid per day might be needed in some cases to lower abnormally high homocysteine levels. The scientists have not proven that lowering the homocysteine level to normal will prevent heart attacks and stroke, however. They believe this because inflammatory cells were found at the site of plaque buildup in arteries of some heart attack victims.

One of the sensitive markers of an inflammation is called the C-reactive protein (CRP).

Dr. Paul Ridker proposes that the CRP is a much more sensitive predictor of a heart attack than lipid screening. At least both tests, along with homocysteine and lipid profiles, should be performed. Furthermore, it is his opinion, and others in his group, that the reason aspirin may prevent heart attacks is because it soothes the inflammation around the plaque. He goes on to explain why some men have heart attacks with normal LDL and cholesterol levels.

Going along with the concept of chronic bacteria infection as the cause of coronary artery disease, some claim periodontal disease and dental caries are associated with increased incidence of cardiovascular and cerebral vascular events. Having no teeth is also a risk factor, they believe.

Of course, it is good hygiene to have clean teeth and

healthy gums. More studies in progress will explore this link-age between bad teeth and heart disease.

New ideas are coming forth each month and, by the time this book lands in the anxious hands of the public, surely new unproven concepts will be bouncing from our TV and Internet screens.

Now if Big Ed, or Willard, had a test for their lipid level in the blood and a homocysteine level, it undoubtedly would have been found to be elevated. Besides starting them on the diet I suggested, I would have prescribed lipid-lowering drug.

I would have urged these men to have an exercise stress test, even if they had normal lipids in their blood, because of the family history of heart disease and the vigorous physical activity they engaged in. Likewise, any smoker, or persons with hypertension and diabetes, should have a stress test.

Diabetic male patients have a two- to three-times-greater chance of a heart attack, especially if they have poor control of their blood sugar. Today, the level of HbA1c in the blood determines control of blood sugar. Good control of diabetes is indicated if the HbA1c is less than 7.3 percent.

The spouse should ask the doctor caring for her man what the level of the HbA1c is and not only what the blood sugar level is.

The stress test: What is it?

"I don't need a stress test, doc, I have enough stress every day on my job, at home, and watching the market," the man said to me, "but my wife insists."

I explained to the patient, named Mac:

"I am going to attach some electrodes to your chest; they are connected to the ECG, and then you will walk on this treadmill. We will gradually increase the speed and the incline until you have reached as near as possible your predicted heart rate, and monitor your ECG. We will stop the test if you feel too tired, get short of breath, or if any tightness or chest pain occurs. We will also stop it if your heart becomes irregular or your blood pressure suddenly falls.

"After you have reached the desired heart rate, you will then lie down on the table and we will continue checking your blood pressure and recording your ECG.

"In addition, in our cardiac laboratory we will get a picture of your heart, called an echocardiogram, before you start exercising and then another right after you come down from the treadmill, to see how your heart behaves. If you have blocked coronary arteries greater than 75 percent it will probably show up on the electrocardiogram, and on the echocardiogram after exercise. We measure your wall motion, which would be impaired if not enough blood arrives to the heart muscle."

"Okay, doc, go ahead, but can I die from this test?" Mac asked me before we got started.

"Good question, Mac. After performing almost 200,000 or more stress tests in the past thirty years, we have not had one person die on the treadmill. Nationwide statistics are about the same. I heard of one lawyer who died on the treadmill recently, but he had chest pain and did not tell anyone. We would not perform this test if someone complains of chest pain at the time of the examination, regardless of the type of pain, until we are certain that person is not having a heart attack."

"How long has this test been around?" Mac asked me.

"Believe it or not, it's about sixty years. Dr. Arthur Master, a well-known cardiologist in New York, devised a simple stress test by having patients run up and down two steps on a ladder, called the two-step test. He performed an ECG before and after; patients' pulse rates increased substantially, and Dr. Master got about the same information we now get from this expensive test."

My nurse, an expert stress test technician, prepared the patient: She first gave him some water to drink, as dehydration can cause the blood pressure to fall and thus skew the test results.

After the patient's chest was exposed, she connected the electrodes to the patient.

The test began. Mac had no symptoms, but his father died at an early age from a heart attack. Mac's LDL was 200, his cholesterol reading was 280, and the HDL was 25. His blood pressure was 150/95. He had stopped smoking several years earlier only because of his spouse's persistence. As a matter of fact, it was because of his wife's insistence that the family doctor sent her husband to see a cardiologist who performs stress tests. She also read that a stress test improperly performed by some commercial clinics with no doctor in attendance could be dangerous.

The HMO turned down the request to perform a stress test on a "healthy man." We urge men and women to have stress tests if their LDL is 200 and HDL is down to 30 or lower. Mac's wife decided it was worth the money to pay "out of pocket" and quit the HMO to join a private insurer. Alas, not all Americans have that privilege.

Mac liked the idea of the treadmill, "A good workout," he said.

There are five stages of standard protocol, with each stage becoming more difficult as the treadmill increases in speed as well as in inclination. By the end of stage 111, Mac became very tired, his heart rate was 138—his predicted goal was

150—and his blood pressure jumped up to 200 systolic and 110 diastolic. The test was stopped because the ECG had changed from the base line, the so-called ST segment dropped, and the echocardiogram showed a large defect on the front of the heart. With these dramatic findings, I urged Mac to be admitted to the hospital for a cardiac catheterization to see how many arteries were blocked and to what extent.

If his stress echocardiogram test was not so significantly positive, Mac could have had another stress test, called a radioisotope, where thallium or technetium 99m-sestamibi, is injected into a vein during the stress test. Areas of the heart not receiving enough blood, called an ischemic area, is readily found by this technique. It has close to a 90 percent accuracy rate.

What is cardiac catheterization?

Mac asked, "Do you mind if my wife Ann hears this explanation, because she can understand this stuff better than I."

A cardiac catheterization means the passage of a tube through a blood vessel in the arm or groin and then into the heart. When a dye is injected into the tube (catheter), it is called coronary angiography. It produces a sort of X-ray of the coronary arteries. It is considered the "Gold Standard," as it gives us accurate information on whether the coronary arteries are diseased, and whether or not the heart valves are functioning correctly.

"Is it safe to have this procedure done?" Mac's wife asked, "and what are the complications?"

The test has few complications, if performed by expert

hands. There may be some bleeding at the site where the catheter is snaked into the thigh. More serious side effects occur in rare instances, however. The catheter may perforate the heart and some plaque may be dislodged, causing a heart attack or stroke. The death rate is extremely low. This procedure is performed at least 800,000 times a year and it gives us a clear picture of what arteries are blocked and by how much. It provides a road map to best plan the most beneficial treatment for the patient.

As a point of interest, a surgeon, Dr. Werner Forssmann, a German scientist, performed the first cardiac catheterization. He studied how tubes could be inserted into the veins and arteries of horses; he concluded that the same might work for man. Secretly, one night, Dr. Forssmann injected a small amount of anesthetic into his arm and then proceeded to snake a long tube into a vein. The catheter was used to pass into the urinary bladder. He was almost interrupted by a colleague, Peter Romas, who came storming into the room screaming, "What the hell are you doing?" Disregarding his colleague's plea, Forssmann placed a mirror in front of a fluoroscope screen and proceeded to snake the tube into his vein. He visualized his own coronary arteries and won the Nobel Prize in medicine in 1956.

Early the following morning, Mac was admitted into the hospital and placed into the modern catheterization laboratory. The groin was prepared and the tubes passed. As Mac watched on the screen, his arteries received the dye. In forty-five minutes or so Mac was back in his room, the films were developed, and I explained the result to Mac and his wife.

"Everything went very well, Mac," I told him, "but you will have to lie still for a while so you don't bleed. We sutured the spot we entered in your thigh, and the chance of a leg artery becoming swollen is slight; that would be called a pseudoaneurism."

"The pictures show you have a major blockage of the important artery called the left anterior descending artery, which supplies most of the blood to the front of the heart. It is actually 98 percent blocked. So, you are lucky we got you in here because if it suddenly blocks 100 percent you can lose most of your heart muscle. The blockage is proximal, and just above the center of the long artery. We can easily open this with an angioplasty, or surgery. I suggest you have an angioplasty, because it is safer, quicker, and you will be out of the hospital in a few days."

"I feel great, doc," Mac said, "why can't I wait and you treat me with medications."

"Not a good idea, Mac, because the chances are very likely you will have a heart attack in the next six months, even with medications. You could die or have such massive heart damage that you will require multiple medications. Your quality of life would be poor and your life span would be dramatically reduced."

This "balloon" treatment, called coronary angioplasty or PTCA (percutaneous transluminal coronary angioplasty), was first performed by Andre Gruntzig who used a balloon catheter in 1977.

According to the National Heart, Lung and Blood Registry, the initial success rate of angioplasty is close to 90 percent. The blockage is reduced from 98 percent to 30 percent. Angioplasty is far from being a panacea, but it saves lives. Unfortunately, there is a 30 percent chance of it closing again within six months. Some have to be redone in forty-eight hours. That number stands at 4 percent. But with the new antiplatelets and stents to keep the arteries open, the success rate is improved. Stents are mesh-like grates placed to keep the artery opened.

One side effect you should be aware of (that occurs in only 5 percent of cases) is that the blocked artery goes into spasm or hemorrhages occur inside of the artery during or after the balloon is placed. Now the artery is blocked 100 percent and emergency surgery must be performed. A heart surgeon must be standing by during the angioplasty.

"Now tell me if you or your wife know of a heart surgeon that we can notify to be on call."

"Can my husband die from this procedure?" Mac's wife asked.

The fatality rate from balloon angioplasty is less than one percent, as it is from bypass surgery.

"I have read of laser treatment, or radiation," his wife said. "What is it?"

The desired area is spot radiated, or laser beams are used. It is still a little too early to make a decision to use these therapies on a routine basis. "If all goes well, and it will, Mac, you will leave the hospital in a few days in a much safer condition than when you arrived."

Mac had a successful balloon angioplasty and came home in a few days. He was given a prescription of 300 mg aspirin, Plavix (clopidrogel), a strong antiplatelet chemical, and the low-fat diet described in this book. His cholesterol and LDL were elevated, and he was given a statin to be taken in the evening. I also included folic acid 2 mg, B12, B6 and an ACE inhibitor for his hypertension. He was encouraged to walk at least one mile four times per week and he could resume all his sexual activity as before. The ACE-inhibitor not only controls hypertension, but also improves the function of endothelium of the artery, and prevents heart attacks and stroke. We give them to patients with normal blood pressure.

One month later, Mac had a repeat exercise stress test and an evaluation of blood lipids. His stress test was now normal, but his LDL did not reach the level of 90 or 80, which is the goal I set for all men who have elevated LDL. One month later, after his statin dosage was doubled, his LDL dropped down to 80 and his HDL rose to 50. Mac will have a stress test every six months for the first year or two. Three years after his operation, Mac is doing just fine.

This is a true story that is repeated dozens and dozens of times each year throughout our country. Mac's life was saved because his spouse was there to guide him. She suggested he take garlic, olive oil, walnuts, and one glass of red wine, with which I fully concurred. Although he had no chest pain or shortness of breath or fatigue, the risk factors were in place to cause a cardiac disaster.

Now the story of Henry, a retired bookie, is a little different. He was having chest pain on and off for years and he placed his bets on medical treatment—and not surgical treatment—with lots of nitroglycerine for his pain (10–12 per day), beta-blockers, aspirin, garlic, Vitamin E, chromium, zinc, St. John's wort, selenium, gingko biloba, and ginseng. He was proud of the fact that he avoided catheterization and, perhaps, surgery. But one fine day, "the gambler" had a fainting episode and did not go to the emergency room but landed right at my door. His ECG was normal, but he was suffering from angina. The bookie consented (with the urging of his girlfriend) to admission to the hospital and he underwent a cardiac catheterization.

The catheterization disclosed that all his three coronary arteries were blocked by 99 percent, and I told him only surgery would save his life. He agreed as a betting man, that the odds favored surgery, and he chose it.

The operation consisted of four bypasses, using an artery from his chest called the internal mammary artery and the veins from his leg.

The operation was a success. The patient survived and his room was packed with flowers from his friends.

After I had finished my training at Yale Medical School, and started practicing in New Haven, I received a call from the Attorney General's office in Washington D.C., asking if I would be willing to see a federal prisoner for a consultation. Doctors from Houston stated that if this outlaw went to prison he would die from the stress because he was suffering from severe coronary artery disease and angina. The Attorney General's office called Yale Medical School to find a doctor to offer a second opinion. I was delighted to be chosen, since I had about five patients in my practice at that time.

Three days later, two strong looking guys who looked like they were borrowed from central casting for an FBI movie, entered my office with a nice young-looking man in handcuffs.

Just at that instant my phone rang and a muffled voice on the other end said simply, "Hey, doc, you are young, just starting out, don't send M to jail." He hung up and M was brought into my examining room. I examined him and he complained of severe angina at rest and while walking. He kept telling me he was only 37 years old, his father and brother died of heart attacks, and if he went to prison in Texas he will surely die.

"You have to save me. The other doctors in Texas said if I go to prison I will be dead in two weeks."

His catheterization results, which came along with his records from Houston, showed all his arteries blocked by 90 percent. Indeed, the hoodlum was very amiable, and I was just a bit uneasy to be the one to make a decision whether going to jail would kill him, especially after that scary phone call. Likewise, these experienced, learned doctors in Houston felt that the stress of imprisonment would kill M.

Here is what I decided in my Talmudic reasoning:

"Listen, Mr. M, you do have terribly blocked arteries and you are in constant danger of sudden death. Your Houston doctors are right about that. But if you don't go to jail you will die sooner. Your lifestyle of drinking, smoking, and hard living will finish you off. My advice to you is to not worry about going to jail. (He gasped in pain.) Once you're there, that world-famous heart surgeon you saw will operate on you, because I am certain you will land in the prison hospital—and the government will pay for the best care. We are a benevolent country even regarding those who break the law."

The hoodlum gave me a "Cheshire cat" smile, as if he swallowed a canary, and agreed that he might be better off in jail instead of pursuing his downtrodden way of life as a free man. He was also influenced by the fact that the best heart surgeon would operate on him free of charge.

This story has a happy ending for M. Hours after he was jailed he complained of severe chest pain and was admitted to St. Luke's Hospital and was operated on by the famous surgeon. One year later, I received three bouquets and a note, "Thanks for the right decision."

R.J., a diabetic who took insulin, had been pretty rigorous about controlling his weight and his sugar level, along with the diligent care he received from his wife. She made certain R.J., who was 67 years old, took his medications for hypertension, a baby aspirin, and a statin for his high cholesterol. She read that medications prescribed for hypertension are desirable for diabetics, like her husband, to prevent kidney damage.

One morning, R.J. complained to his wife of feeling very tired and short of breath just walking to the bathroom. His wife did not waste one minute, but called 911 and R.J. was brought to the emergency room. She knew from her readings that diabetics could have heart attacks without complaining of chest pain, but just shortness of breath.

R.J. had an abnormal ECG when he arrived at the emergency room. He was admitted and it turned out he did have a heart attack. Before leaving the hospital, he had a stress test, which came back abnormal and cardiac catheterization showed two arteries were blocked. During that same hospital stay, a balloon angioplasty was performed and R.J. went home after a successful opening of his blocked arteries.

Besides classical chest pain, shortness of breath can be a warning bell that the artery to the heart may be blocked. In this age of asthma and lung ailments, it is not always an easy task to find the cause of shortness of breath. Once again, the spouse should ask questions of the doctor. She could ask, "Can the shortness of breath be a heart attack, because of a lack of oxygen getting to his heart muscle?"

Before a heart attack has actually occurred, his lungs may fill up with water from a weakened heart; this is called congestive heart failure.

"He had indigestion all night, after a few drinks following a spicy Malaysian meal, but I still want to be sure it's not his heart." This is what Agnes told me about her husband over the phone.

"Well, bring him right in," I told her, "he does have a cholesterol problem, and he still smokes."

"He went to work—he would not listen to me," she continued.

"Well get him on the phone; go down to his office and bring him right here, or take him to the emergency room."

Agnes did just that. She picked up her husband and, reluctantly, he went along with being driven to a local emergency room near his workplace. The doctor on call diagnosed Agnes' husband as having sustained a large heart attack of the front of his heart, called an anterior myocardial infarction. He survived and, in the future, will need a cardiac catheterization to get a picture of his arteries to see if they can be opened with a balloon, or by use of a stent, or, if indicated, have surgery.

Indigestion and heartburn can be very common symptoms of a heart attack, even if the person is known to have chronic regurgitation of acid—called esophageal reflux or GERD—and is taking antacids. Years ago the newspaper would report the sudden death of a person dying of indigestion.

This is another difficult problem for the doctor: to distinguish between heartburn and a heart attack. Again, I implore the wife to ask the doctor, "Are you sure it is not his heart?" The doctor then, in turn, will perform tests already discussed, to make certain it is not a heart attack or angina.

To summarize, your should be aware if your spouse has any of the following problems:

1. He is a smoker
2. He has high LDL
3. He is overweight
4. He has a strong family history of heart attacks and death
5. He has been feeling fatigued more than usual
6. He has high blood pressure

7. He has diabetes
8. He has a homocysteine level, above 10
9. He has peripheral vascular insufficiency (poor circulation in the legs)

All the above increase risk rates for a heart attack and, thus, the spouse needs to be vigilant, and she should learn CPR.

If any of the symptoms I have discussed are present—chest pain, shortness of breath, heartburn, weakness and fainting spells—these should alert the spouse to bring her man to a doctor. Your man should have a cardiac stress test once a year if he has the above risk factors.

PERIPHERAL VASCULAR DISEASE (PVD)

There are millions of men suffering from peripheral vascular disease, especially when they are smokers (or former smokers).

Pains in the calf muscles, occurring while walking and then relieved by rest, is a clear sign of poor circulation. It could mean the arteries in the legs are blocked. It is a serious signal that should also alert a good doctor that the coronary arteries have a 35 to 40 percent chance of being blocked. The arteries leading to the brain, called the carotid arteries, may also be blocked.

The diagnosis of PVD is easily made by a doctor who specializes in PVD, a vascular surgeon or an internist who performs peripheral vascular testing. It is important for the spouse to see that these studies are done when her husband complains of leg pains. In this case, the spouse should ask the examining doctor, "Were my husband's arteries tested both at rest and when he exercises?"

This is important because a resting doppler examination of the arteries can be normal, but exercise on a treadmill can detect poor circulation of the legs if the doppler examination is properly performed before exercise and right after.

THE HEART ATTACK

When I was a newly trained intern in New York City decades ago, I took care of my first heart attack patient. He was 53 years old and he had severe tightness in his chest; he also was sweating profusely. His wife just knew her husband was having a heart attack, as the symptoms were the same when her father suffered a fatal myocardial infarction.

At that time we had no coronary care unit or intensive care unit to treat heart attack patients. All we could do was to place him in an oxygen tent, administer morphine for his pain, and do lots of hand wringing. We watched the man go into cardiac arrest, and administered adrenaline-like drugs as his blood pressure fell. We could do little else and the man died.

Now, only 40 years later, an incredible, miraculous, and far different picture exists today. We can save most men from dying of a heart attack if they arrive at the hospital soon enough.

If your spouse has tightness in his chest, and is perspiring, and fits the risk factors mentioned above, call 911, and give him a regular aspirin, not a coated one (as a coated one takes too long to dissolve). At this point I strongly urge you to know in advance what hospital he can be taken to and, if you live in the suburbs, make sure that the ambulance knows where your home is. If not, have directions ready to be given. More than once it has happened that an ambulance had trouble finding a home and there was a critical delay in treatment.

Speed is of the utmost importance. Once in the hospital, the doctors on call, with the help of a cardiologist, will determine if the man is having a myocardial infarction. They then will decide if he should be given a clot buster called TPA (for thrombolysis) or go directly to the catheterization laboratory, if one is available, and perform an angioplasty to open his blocked artery. If the heart attack occurred more than six to eight hours before, the cardiologist may decide not to perform either of the procedures, but admit your spouse for a few days and observe him. They will most likely perform a stress test before discharging him, and likely prescribe a cardiac catheterization to see how many arteries are blocked.

Other atypical symptoms of a heart attack are abdominal pain, gastrointestinal distress, changes in mental status, weakness, arrhythmia, and stroke. There are also "silent" heart attacks that have no apparent symptoms at all, except those that the doctor will find on an ECG. Tragically, sudden death may be the first sign of a heart attack.

Today we could save more lives from heart attacks with the help of the spouse, especially if she plans in advance what she would do to help her husband. I also urge the partner to learn CPR, which today involves simple hand pumping of the chest and does not require mouth-to-mouth breathing. The Red Cross and the Emergency Medical technician folks offer CPR courses in almost all communities.

The Heimlich maneuver, another life-saving maneuver, should be learned by the spouse to prevent sudden death of her husband. This is a method of squeezing the chest to extract a foreign object stuck in the laryngopharynx. If not ejected, sudden death from choking can follow.

Are there other causes of impending disaster that are present with chest pain, which are not caused by a heart attack?

Be aware: if the emergency room doctor says that your spouse suffered no heart attack, you should ask about causes of his chest pains. These could include:

1. aortic dissection (aorta suddenly tearing)
2. myocarditis (infection of the heart)
3. collapsed lung, called a pneumothorax
4. embolism

SEX—AFTER A HEART ATTACK

It is rare to suffer a heart attack during or after sexual activity. Most of the time it is the wife who fears that if she gets her man too excited he will die in her arms. Having an orgasm will not harm the heart, if anything, it might relax your partner much more than any sedative, once the act is finished.

There have been some reliable studies done that have shown, whether you have a habitual partner or a new one, that the blood pressure and pulse rise during sex is insignificant, unless your blood pressure is very labile. A sudden rise of blood pressure, which is dangerous, can be diagnosed by a treadmill test, and should be treated, regardless of sexual or other physical activity.

How long should you wait after a heart attack or bypass operation to have sex?

If your spouse can climb a flight of stairs without having chest pain, or his pulse does not rise above 130, you can safely engage in sexual activities with your doctor's approval.

Can he use Viagra after a heart attack?

The answer is probably yes! Providing you don't use any nitroglycerine pills or nitroglycerine patches, as these products can drop the blood pressure to a dangerous level when used with Viagra. Ask your doctor before you resume using Viagra or starting it for the first time.

Sex is a terrific exercise; it beats the boring treadmill. Depending on how you and your partner go about it, up to ten calories per minute or more are burned during sexual intercourse.

HYPERTENSION

Neglected high blood pressure, either systolic (upper number) or diastolic (lower number), is a major cause of strokes, congestive heart failure and heart attacks.

In men over the age of 55, the systolic blood pressure reading should be below 135, as mentioned earlier, especially if these men are suffering from diabetes.

The spouse once more can be of great help in saving her husband's life, so he can live as long as she does. She should obtain a good reliable blood pressure monitor and have her doctor check its accuracy. She then can become an active participant in the control of the blood pressure of her spouse. This also avoids running to the doctor to have the blood pressure checked.

Nighttime reading of blood pressure can be very important, especially if her man takes medications to control blood pressure; if the nighttime readings reveal systolic pressure above 140 or 150, the treating doctor should be consulted to make the appropriate adjustments.

More than 60 percent of men over the age of 60 have hypertension, and I suspect many of these men do not have good blood pressure control. Blood pressure readings differ from hour to hour, and even from minute to minute. A blood pressure reading taken in a doctor's office once a month or more does not tell the entire story. What is the difference between blood pressure during the day and during the night? These are questions that the spouse frequently should address.

Most blood pressure measurements and treatment are done by the family doctor, and it is the most common malady treated by a general practitioner. It is highly complicated and difficult to properly treat hypertension, since, as of today, there are no ideal medications available to treat it. Side effects abound and, although mild to be sure, they discourage the patient from taking the available medications. The goals of good blood control are hard to achieve with one drug—often it requires prescriptions of two or more drugs.

Because so much information is given to the person taking blood pressure pills, a form of drug paranoia emerges regarding possible side effects. Any symptoms that arise after the pill is started "must be due to the drug."

All doctors have the same misadventures in treating high blood pressure. Difficulties occur because of the cost of the medications and the tight-fisted HMOs who will pay for drug "A," but not for drug "B." It becomes a constant source of frustration for the patient, the doctor, and the pharmacist when the an HMO refuses to pay for a drug with which the doctor is most familiar, and with which he has had the most experience and the best results.

The HMO often requires a special letter from the attending physician justifying why he feels the patient should have that particular medication. Obviously, the HMO wants the cheapest drug to be used, and they know damn well that the doctor has little time to write letters justifying his reasons for prescribing a specific drug. Phone calls from the patient and the pharmacy then follow, and soon the doctor will need to be treated for hypertension!

All these factors combine to create one of the major reasons for poor blood pressure control. We must not forget to mention that the patient often gets lost in this thicket and stops the medication on his own; when the bottle is finished the blood pressure pill is not renewed because of cost. Patients justify this by saying, "I did not think I had to continue to take the blood pressure pills."

Now here again, the spouse on the white horse can come to the rescue: "Please dear, I love you, and I don't want you to have a stroke. We need you, so get the prescription filled and let's make an appointment with Dr. Y to see how you are doing."

PALPITATIONS

Palpitations are unusual heart rhythms, such as skipped heartbeats, extra heartbeats, extrasystole, rapid heartbeats, rapid irregular heartbeats, slow pulse, atrial fibrillation, and ventricular tachycardia. All are "palpitations" that can be responsible for sudden death. These heartbeats can occur with normal coronary arteries and normal heart muscle.

Some irregular heart rhythms are potentially dangerous, and others are merely ongoing nuisances—frightening, but not dangerous to your husband's life.

Note well, however, that all palpitations need to be investigated to determine their cause (and treatment, if needed).

Many times abnormal heartbeats can arise from too much alcohol, cigarettes, caffeine, or too many anxious moments. Once these elements are eliminated, it can solve the problem of the abnormal heartbeat.

Atrial fibrillation is a very common disorder that has many causes, from narrowed coronary arteries, abnormal valve, to "alcohol heart," and is an especially common disorder in men over the age of 65.

Here again, the spouse can help avert a catastrophe by assisting her husband in regulating the blood thinner, Coumadin, often given for atrial fibrillation. The INR is the test used to determine how thin the blood is. If it is too high above (4.0), bleeding can occur in the brain, or, perhaps, somewhere else. If it is too low (below 1.8), the blood thinner does not work; a clot can form, travel to the brain, and result in a stroke. Blood thinner is the current remedy in preventing a stroke inpatients who suffer from atrial fibrillation.

Recently, self-testing by the patient with machines that measure the INR have become available. These machines are especially useful to men who are homebound or, because of bad weather conditions, or distances from test sites, are unable to have their blood tests. In Europe, these machines have become quite popular and Europeans have been shown to have a much safer margin by self-testing than going to a standing laboratory. Patients forget to go, or just skip their tests, which can result in poor control and cause hemorrhages in the brain, or, on the contrary, have no anti-coagulation and suffer strokes. Patients must be educated as to what pills not to take, which can make them vulnerable to bleeding, and even foods such as broccoli and other green salads that can interfere with proper control of their INR. As mentioned in other chapters, certain medications can interfere with the action of Coumadin. The spouse should ask her husband's doctor if the medications or herbs her man is taking cross-react with Coumadin. For example, Coumadin and Prilosec sometimes interact, making the INR too high.

Even today, with all the information available, the majority of patients suffering from atrial fibrillation are not receiving Coumadin to prevent a stroke.

The aim of treatment for atrial fibrillation is to control the heart rate, lest it becomes too fast. If it does, it can weaken the patient and the heart muscle as well. The treatment of atrial fibrillation is not an easy matter. It requires a cardiologist or experienced internist to manage this complex condition.

As men age, the electrical conducting system in their hearts can degenerate and cause slowing of conduction, slow heartbeats, which may result in a complete heart block, fainting spells, and death.

The miracle of the pacemaker, first discovered in 1872 by Dr. Armand Duchene, was first used on the outside of the chest. In November 1956, Dr. Henry Bahnson of Johns

Hopkins University placed electrodes inside the chest, for the first internal pacemaker. Dr. Walter Lilleihei, also from Johns Hopkins University, continued the work and brought pacemakers to the forefront of cardiology.

If your spouse complains of palpitations, he should receive the following in addition to a thorough physical examination:

1. ECG
2.. Holter monitor or event monitor
3. Echocardiogram to see his heart valves
4. May need a stress test
5. Thyroid blood tests
6. May need to see expert on heart rhythm—and have electrical conduction test

THE ULTRAFAST SCAN

"My neighbor said there is a new test to see if the coronary arteries are blocked," said the wife one day. "I read it in the local paper. It's called the Ultrafast Scan. What is that?"

The ultrafast scan (EBCT), also called the electron beam CAT scan, is not a new test; it merely measures the amount of calcium present in the coronary arteries. "Nothing new under the sun," one sage said, and how true it is. We have been detecting calcium in the coronary arteries by fluoroscopy for at least sixty years.

This test costs around $500 dollars, and it takes just a few minutes to perform. It determines if you have a significant amount of calcium in your arteries. There are calcium scores that show up when measured by an experienced radiologist with this technique; it allegedly predicts if the patient is prone to heart attack.

At a recent American College of Cardiology meeting, this topic was thoroughly examined. The conclusions, although controversial, stated the presence of calcium in the arteries is a marker for arteriosclerosis or plaque, but there is not enough proof that it can predict a heart attack.

In my opinion, having no plaque is a good thing, but most people over the age of 55 will have some plaque, and this may not be a bad thing. If plaque is present, it is a hard plaque and will, therefore, be stable. Plaque that is stable does not crack easily and allow a potentially dangerous clot to form. The issue is not the plaque but, rather, whether there is an impediment to the flow of blood through the coronary arteries. If your man has no symptoms and no risk factors, I don't advise him to spend the money to discover the presence of calcium in the arteries.

Also on the horizon, are techniques being developed to visualize the coronary arteries, without having to perform cardiac catheterization using magnetic resonance (MRI) techniques.

PREVENTION IS THE BEST WAY to avoid a heart attack. Both you and your spouse should follow the recommendations I have made in this book.

In summary, the spouse is like a surrogate doctor for her husband who can do much to save her husband from sudden death, if her husband is willing to cooperate with her—and that is where the real problem lies.

Chapter Nine

What the Doctor Missed During Your Husband's Annual Physical

I WROTE A TEXTBOOK that was published in 1987, entitled *Physical Diagnosis for Medical Students,* and the foreword was written by one of the most prominent men of science—Professor Alvan Feinstein of the Yale University School of Medicine. He wrote: "This book will also be of interest to medical historians in the future." How perceptive this doctor was!

Physical diagnosis is the very art and foundation of the practice of medicine. It is the tools of our trade. For hundreds of years, by using our senses—sharp eyes and ears, gentle touching hands, and our educated brains—we could make most diagnoses without the need of thousands of tests.

Thousands of years ago, Hippocrates, the father of medicine, while teaching medicine to his students on the Isle of Kos, in Greece, said the following:

"A great part, I believe, of the art is to be able to observe. Leave nothing to chance. Overlook nothing. Study the patient, rather than the disease."

Hippocrates also said, "Life is short and the art is long." The art of deduction, the brilliance of our forefathers with their ingenious intuition, and a Sherlock Holmes–like sense of detection based on observation is much needed in today's medicine.

Prior to the great French physician Laennec, who discovered the stethoscope, doctors would listen to the heart by placing a napkin on the naked chest of the female and place his ear directly on the chest to hear sounds of the heart.

Gustav Mahler, the Great Austrian composer, wrote that after hearing part of a symphony, one night lying in bed, his own heart transmitted the ominous sounds of his sick heart muscle called a gallop rhythm—the triple beat that sounds like the gallop of a horse.

The stethoscope, the very mark of the medical doctor, has become a relic of medicine. It hangs around the neck or dangles from the side pocket but it no longer has the power of a diagnostic tool as it once did. Listening to the heart, called auscultation, is no longer formally taught in most medical schools on an individual basis. I know, because I used to be one of the teachers.

On July 13, 1999, *The New York Times* reported: "Educators are startled by and unhappy with these trends, particularly since the physical examination can also be a technique for effectively controlling health care costs."

Physicians are losing their skills and their judgments on their findings, and thus swiftly turn to the tests for diagnosis. Students spend more time with computers than with patients. Doctors in practice are forced to spend ten times more time on paperwork and less and less time with the patient. Nurses spend more time on keeping proper notes on the patient rather than at bedside caring for the patient.

We health workers are judged *not* by how well our patients do, or the effort and time we spend with the patient, but how neat and clean are the pages full of notes that the despotic HMOs and Medicare base their decisions on for reimbursement.

I have asked insurance carriers to interview patients and learn from those patients just how good and honest, or poor, the doctor's performance is, rather than wasting hours upon hours on chart reviews.

Everything we do in our society is swift and quick, and the practice of medicine also is a victim of this hurried frenzy. Patients expect quick answers and fast results; both constitute unreasonable expectations.

Because of encouragement by the government over the last eight years, insurance companies and managed care have taken control over the practice of medicine. Lawyers have forced doctors to do too many tests, many of which are unnecessary. Woe to the doctor who failed to perform a test that later turns out to be necessary. To avoid the malpractice suit the doctor will order tests even if in his judgment they are most likely going to yield nothing.

But if there is a small, remote chance that the test will be positive, the doctor will suffer many years of humiliation and sleepless nights. We are a litigious society; patients and lawyers have discovered a windfall of money. "Don't take it personally, doctor, let the insurance company pay; that is why you have insurance," so said one lawyer to a doctor.

In Europe, malpractice is rare and the art of physical diagnosis still flourishes. Our medical system, as judged by the World Health Organization in a recent survey, ranks 39th in the world, while France is number one.

The government, insurance companies, and the legal profession have helped to bring on this downward spiral of a doctor's physical diagnosis skills. Ask any doctor in practice or teacher in medical school and they will agree that the physical diagnosis skills have atrophied. I fear our new generation of doctors has also become victim to our new medical care—the inability to diagnose a heart ailment with only a stethoscope after taking a thorough history of the patient.

A good history taken from the patient is the very essence of arriving at a diagnosis before any tests are performed. Medical students used to read *The Adventures of Sherlock Holmes* to see how Holmes made deductions based on small clues that seemed like insufficient evidence. The creator of Sherlock Holmes, Sir Arthur Conan Doyle, was a physician.

A good history takes time, and time is no longer amply allotted to the practicing doctor. The well-trained, experienced clinician gets clues from the very appearance of the patient. The manner in which the patient walks, talks, the color of his eyes (e.g., are they tinged yellow as in hepatitis?), and his voice (is it hoarse like that of a smoker?), are all important.

More often than not, patients will demand CAT scans, MRIs and new tests that appeared on the six o'clock news or in *The Wall Street Journal*, and not trust the doctor's judgment.

There is another side to the story—a despairing one, I might add. In June of 2000, in Milwaukee, the American Society of Hypertension released a study that found 95 out of 100 medical students, after a one-year course on how to take a patient's blood pressure, were doing it incorrectly.

At the prestigious Duke University Medical Center in Durham, North Carolina, another study showed that the residents were only 50 percent accurate when listening to patients with damaged heart valves.

What, then, should the patient expect from the doctor performing an annual physical examination? The physician should spend the time to get an accurate medical and surgical history and review at least the medical form that the patient filled out. It should include a family history, smoking and alcohol history, and information on allergies. Today it is common practice to get sexual preference history, detailing sexual habits including the use of condoms. Today, AIDS is one of our most dreaded diseases and is running rampant in men and women. The doctor should inquire discreetly about the patient's relationship with his spouse and children.

Recently, one female patient of mine was upset because I never asked her if she was sexually abused. "You should have asked me that ten years ago," she said. Again I learned something from a patient. My generation rarely discussed sexual matters in a family practice. Until recently we now inquire if the man is impotent and many times they lie to us because they are too embarrassed—especially the strict conservative types.

A brief psychiatric evaluation should be performed, which includes a sleep history, an evaluation of mood swings, and basic questions regarding their work and family relationships.

The examining doctor should spend some time obtaining a dietary history. He should get a list of all medications the spouse takes and all the alternative herbs and devices the patient uses daily, as well as the type of exercise in which he indulges.

THE PHYSICAL EXAMINATION

Blood Pressure Measurements. It should not be taken as soon as you come into the doctor's office. The patient should sit for five minutes before the nurse or doctor performs the readings, either, because the blood pressure may be elevated just from the physical activity of coming into the office. Coffee should be avoided at least one hour before blood pressure readings are taken.

It is incorrect to take the blood pressure over any clothing, and if the arm is fat a larger cuff has to be used because erroneous elevated readings can result.

The blood pressure readings can vary from minute to minute, and three readings are needed on the right and left arm. The patient should be standing for a few minutes and measurements then taken. As in some patients, a marked fall in blood pressure can be a cause of dizziness.

If the blood pressure is found elevated greater than 135/85 three readings should be done on three separate days.

Examination of the Mouth and Nose. The doctor will inspect the tonsils (if present), and the color of the mucous to see if it is pale or anemic. Years ago, the doctor looked for a blue line on the gums that signaled lead poisoning.

Examination of the nose is to look for collapse of the septum, found in cocaine users.

Heart Examination. The stethoscope should be used on the naked chest and not through a shirt as I have seen some professionals do. The doctor will listen to the sounds of the heart over the valve areas with the patient lying flat, then turned to the left and, finally, sitting forward.

Ask the examining doctor: "Do you hear a murmur or any other unusual heart sounds?"

Examination of the Lungs. The doctor should ask you to take deep and full breaths in order to hear the normal and abnormal lung sounds such as rales and wheezes. Asthma has increased dramatically and can be detected with the stethoscope. But the rule in medicine is: "All that wheezes is not asthma." It can be a sign of heart failure.

Examination of the Abdomen. The doctor will palpate the abdomen to feel the size of the liver and spleen and then examine each quadrant of the abdomen, looking for masses. He should try to feel for the abdominal aorta to see if it is enlarged. An aneurysm can sometimes be felt by an examiner and save the life of a patient.

If you have a family history of an aneurysm, ask the doctor to double-check you. He should get a CAT scan of the abdomen.

Examination of the Extremities. In examining the extremities the doctor will move, bend, and raise up your arms, elbows, wrists, fingers, hips, knees, and ankles to see if there are any deformities or pain.

The Neurological Examination. With a neurological hammer the reflexes of the upper and lower extremities should be tested—including muscle strength. The cranial nerves, all twelve of them, should be checked. Sensory perception of the upper and lower extremities are also tested.

Checking the Vascular System. The pulses should be checked:

In the neck, the carotid should be checked. On both arms, the brachial and radial should be tested at the wrists.

In the thighs, the femoral arteries should be checked; in the calves, the pedial arteries on the top of the foot and the tibial arteries on the inside of the ankle should be looked at. The artery in the crux of the knee (called the poplitial artery) is difficult to find even by the experts.

The artery examinations are crucial because absence of pulsation in the carotid arteries can signal that a stroke can occur if the carotid arteries are blocked. The stethoscope should be used to examine the carotid arteries in the neck to listen to sounds called "bruits." (How many times has your doctor placed his stethoscope on the neck to listen for bruits?)

If the leg arteries are blocked, the blockage can cause impotence and loss of the legs. It may also be a distant sign of an impending obstruction of the coronary arteries.

The veins of the legs should be examined for the presence of varicose veins, which will alert the patient that he can form clots that can travel to the lung to cause a pulmonary embolism and death. This almost happened to me!

The Rectal Examination. Hopefully, the examiner can perform a gentle examination and feel for prostate size and smoothness, and at the same time take a stool sample to test for blood.

Prior to the use of PSA examinations, doctors attempted to diagnose cancer of the prostate solely by feeling the prostate.

This is a brief and a superficial outline of how a physical examination should be performed. Your spouse should expect all the things I have described; if he receives less, change doctors. I know I did when I had my physical examination a few years ago.

HOW ABOUT THE TESTS?

An Electrocardiogram. After reading electrocardiograms over thirty-eight years, too many to count, I found that most ECGs are normal. Unfortunately, today's computer reading performed for the family doctors often gives a false reading and, I know from experience, at times an abnormal computer reading can actually be a variation of a normal. Generalists will check with a cardiologist if an abnormal reading comes through.

Basic Blood Tests. (to be performed for a routine physical) If the patient has symptoms, blood samples will be taken according to what organ or illness the doctor is trying to discover. Otherwise, routine tests should include:

- Blood count
- Kidney tests
- Liver tests
- Lipid profile
- PSA for men over 40

If I had my way, I would perform a routine test for AIDS instead of the routine tests for syphilis, which is still a prerequisite in most states for a marriage license. I have asked patients if they want an AIDS test, and most say, "I don't need one." Doctors cannot perform tests for AIDS without written consent from the patient.

If the man over 40 has a strong family history of heart disease, I will recommend a cardiac exercise stress test and a colonoscopy if there is a family history of cancer of the colon. Ideally, for a man 55 or older, I would do routine stress tests every four years and a colonoscopy every five to eight years.

I want to administer the same tests to my patients on a yearly basis—the same timetable that is used by the White House physicians attending the president and other highly-placed individuals in both the public and private sectors. We Americans should demand that from our doctors and our insurance carriers. Treat us like the president. We are hard-working Americans, as good as both the leader of our country and the CEO of the pharmaceutical companies. Don't you agree?

Chapter Ten

The Alzheimer's Epidemic: Recognizing the Earliest Symptoms

IN 1982, I SURVIVED a midair plane crash. A fire swept through the plane and the burning inferno crashed into a partially frozen reservoir in Rhode Island. By some miracle, I was only minimally injured, except the hair on my head was seared and it became gray overnight.

For weeks thereafter, I had moments when I would forget my home phone number, the driving directions to my office, and I suffered serious short-term memory loss.

The doctors felt that this was from the smoke inhalation, as I did become unconscious, and suddenly woke up from the impact of the crash. Two others on this small commuter plane, flying from New Haven to Boston were not so lucky.

My medical consultants feared I was going to have permanent memory loss resulting from the plane crash. "Early Alzheimers," one said. It was discovered that the airline's gross negligence caused the fire in midair, but my lawyers cautioned me not to sue the airline. My only injury was memory loss; the publicity that would follow would have put an end to my very active medical career.

One month later my memory returned and I was able to do rapid calculation and solve problems from my old algebra and calculus books, as well as solve chemical formulas from my quantitative analysis and organic chemistry books. Most pleasing, of course, was my ability to recite from memory the "To be or not to be," soliloquy from *Hamlet*; indeed, my memory fully returned in two months.

That episode of memory loss was the impetus to write a book entitled, *Aging Myths: Reversible Causes of Mind and Memory Loss.*

After the age of 50 or so, loss of memory was once called the beginning of senility as a consequence of aging. Today, we recognize that severe memory loss is not always due to aging, but sometimes is caused by a disease or a traumatic event, as it was in my case.

Aging is not an illness, but illness can cause early aging and memory loss. Impairment of intellectual capacity (which includes memory loss, cognition, language, and daily skills) results from brain degeneration, now called *dementia*. There are numerous causes for dementia, which include medications, dozens of illnesses, and the most common one, Alzheimer's disease.

If the spouse begins to notice her mate is becoming forgetful, she should not attribute it to "getting older." There are many medical conditions that cause memory loss and, once treated, the memory can improve.

Depression is a common cause for memory loss, called pseudodementia. Depression may also be an early symptom of dementia.

The tragedy of early onset of memory loss may first become evident only at home. It becomes a family secret. At work, if he is an executive, his entourage will likely blame it on being distracted; in academia, he will be termed an "absent minded professor."

The spouse will notice subtle changes and she, too, will find rationalization for the husband's onset of memory failure, blaming too much work, not enough sleep, and too many martinis. The latter is one of the many horrors of our society—alcoholism affects at least ten percent of our nation and many are left with a defective brain. Too much alcohol is an appalling poison for the brain. Ask any state trooper at the scene of a fatal accident or attend an AA meeting for the shocking evidence.

"You forgot we had a dinner date with the Browns. How could you? They are our oldest friends," is one of many examples that should alert the spouse that something might be awry with her husband's memory.

The neat, compulsive male can become sloppy and forget where he placed important papers, his car keys, or where he parked his car. He may have forgotten the name of a restaurant they have been going to for years, the names of old friends and familiar places, or he may repeat something to himself over and over again. All can be signs of a catastrophic event occurring in the brain, if the forgetfulness is severe and progressive. The onset of depression in an active male who has no obvious cause may be one of the early signs of Alzheimer's disease.

As time goes on, it becomes more evident to the wife that her husband is not just suffering from mild memory loss as all of us do to some degree as we age. Most people who have some short-term memory loss have no trouble with long-term retrieval. Short-term memory, for example, is forgetting the name of someone whom we've just met or a movie we have just seen. Short-term memory loss is very common and benign, but sometimes it can signal the beginning of brain degeneration.

Although it has been estimated that by the age of ninety, approximately 60 percent of our brain cells are gone, it is the location of these nerve cells that is important. In normal persons, areas involved with memory and intelligence arc spared. If cells are destroyed in the seat of memory—the hippocampus (which looks like a sea horse located in the brain)—both short- and long-term memory loss ensue.

Years ago, the former senior executive of a large company consulted me for a heart problem. His wife called in advance and asked me to check his memory, which was of greater concern to her than his heart.

Bill was his usual charming self and it became evident that he was trying to hide his severe memory loss. It was a presidential election year and I asked Bill who he thought would win. Bill answered, "It's the same old guys, and the same guy who is president now."

"Bill," I asked, "what is the name of the president?"

"You got me there, doc, I forgot."

Bill was 59 years old and a very active man. A few years later, he progressed to full-blown Alzheimer's disease. At that time, we had no medication available for the treatment of Alzheimer's disease as we have today.

Former president Reagan now has advanced Alzheimer's disease, but only his wife probably knows for sure when his illness began.

A very thorough medical examination should be performed to try to find a cause for early brain failure. Too often, memory loss remains a family secret for too long; testing is delayed and, then, treatment may not reverse memory loss.

The patient knows if his memory is failing and, sometimes, will not admit it, even to his doctor. Now, since managed care rules the day, medical privacy no longer exists; anything written in the medical charts is open season for Medicare and insurance companies. All doctors' charts are periodically inspected by insurance personnel, just like in a police state. So if the doctor writes "memory loss" on the chart, dozens upon dozens of people will read it. When we sign up for medical insurance, at the same time we relinquish our privacy because we sign a paper giving the insurance company and the Medicare people the right to inspect our medical charts.

Not so for the people who run our government. President Reagan's brain failure was kept a secret for a very long time. Indeed, other leaders of the world have that privacy: Marshall Pidzucky, the president of Poland, suffered from severe dementia, as did President Woodrow Wilson. The list goes on and on, including the late President Kennedy, who had multiple illnesses, and was given Dexadrine, which he received from the late (and discredited) Dr. Max Jacobsen in New York.

The man who loses his memory knows that if someone finds out, his career is finished. This may be one of the reasons that loss of memory is called the "silent epidemic."

Every organ in the body, once seriously impaired, can cause memory loss. For example, small strokes caused by long-standing hypertension or blocked arteries of the brain can result in destruction of vital memory areas of the brain, like the hippocampus. Doctors call this condition multiinfarction dementia (MID), which can be diagnosed with an MRI.

Medications have a notorious reputation for causing memory impairment; whether it is pills and nose spray bought over the counter, or medications prescribed by your doctor, such as beta-blockers and some antidepressants.

Early diagnosis of Alzheimer's disease is very difficult; even expert neurologists cannot always be 100 percent certain. As mentioned above, severe depression can mimic Alzheimer's disease. The depressed male, when asked who is president of the United States, will answer, "Don't bother me with that stupid question, who cares." The patient suffering from Alzheimer disease might say, "You know, it's the same old guy as always." These patients will try to disguise their loss of memory, sometimes in a shrewd manner. They will substitute words, even create their own language because they lost their linguistic command.

As time goes by, this appalling affliction will make the person almost a mute because they will have forgotten the names of everything they have known before. All the basic human skills such as using a fork or knife, or dressing, will disappear. These afflicted persons are aware of their memory loss and that remorseless progression. Some patients hallucinate and become belligerent, which becomes a colossal challenge to the family, physicians, and caretakers.

Alzheimer's disease, first described by Dr. Alois Alzheimer in 1907, afflicts ten percent of Americans over the age of 65. As of today, there are more than four million persons suffering from this illness and, as we grow older, the numbers will continue to increase. It is the fourth leading cause of death, behind heart disease, cancer, and stroke.

The cause remains a mystery except in some cases where there is a herititary linkage. For example, there is an Arab village in Israel called Wadi Ara where 20 percent of the villagers over the age of 65 have Alzheimer's disease and 60 percent over the age of 85 have the disease, compared to 40 percent generally. Neurologists suggest that a recessive gene, carried by both parents, is responsible.

There are some specific pharmacological treatments available that can help keep the illness somewhat in check. Many neurologists feel the earlier the medication is started, the more effective will be the results. For example, a medication called donepezil may have long-term benefits. Another drug called memantine, used in Germany, slows moderately severe Alzheimer's disease. Vitamin E is currently advised in medical texts to help control this disease.

There is worldwide research being conducted to find the cause and treatment for Alzheimer's disease. Scientists know that the brain of Alzheimer's patients becomes packed with a substance called beta amyloid. Today, clinical trials are underway, using a vaccine to rid the brain of these brown amyloid plaques. This trial will soon be completed.

Advice to the spouse: If your husband is suffering from memory loss, insist upon a thorough diagnostic testing and, if his disease is diagnosed as Alzheimer's disease, there is much hope because research is going on at a feverish pace.

Above all: Get a bracelet for him with his name and phone number, as patients with Alzheimer's disease wander off, sometimes never to be found again. Some estimates conclude that up to 40,000 Alzheimer's patients get lost each year and are never found.

Chapter Eleven

The Depressed Male—
A Common Missed Diagnosis

ONE SATURDAY AFTERNOON, Hendrix showed me his gun collection and shooting gallery in the basement of his luxurious home. His wife, Irene, and my former wife, were good friends. We dined together that same night and almost immediately I had the feeling that all was not well in the Hendrix family.

One week later, Irene called to inform us that Hendrix had died cleaning his .38 caliber gun. The police concluded that it was an accident. Secretly, we learned from Irene that Hendrix probably committed suicide; he had been depressed for years. He had been seeing a chiropractor that was giving him enemas, massages, manipulations, and herbs for back pain.

This is an especially tragic story because perhaps it could have been avoided if Hendrix had psychiatric care. Irene had tried to coax her husband to seek professional help. But Hendrix was too proud and too ashamed to admit to anyone that he was suffering from severe depression. "It would hurt my business if someone found out," he once opined.

My friend Jimmy was an attorney and outwardly a jovial, generous gentleman, who was loved and respected in his community. He suffered from severe depression for years, according to his wife's conversation at the funeral.

Jimmy shot himself in the head one Sunday morning. He was a good actor and he fooled me. I never knew or suspected he was depressed. If his wife had only informed me, perhaps I would have been able to help Jimmy. He came to see me each year to have his heart examined, since his father and grandfather both died of heart attacks.

On the questionnaire we give to patients are the following questions:

Do you ever feel depressed? Have a sleep problem? Are you unable to concentrate? Lost interest in sex? Sports? Or your business? Are things not going well at home or at work? Have you lost your appetite? Are you more tired than usual? Do you wish you were away from it all? Do you wish you were dead? Do you ever think of suicide?

Jimmy had answered "no" to all of these questions.

In many a clinician's office, as well as in mine, the patients sometimes refuse to honestly answer the medical questionnaire. Often, men tell my medical assistant, "I just filled this out last year; I don't have the time for this." Sometimes, the less educated patients may have difficulty reading, or understanding, the questions; some actually are illiterate. They will say, "I don't have my glasses, let me take it home and I will send the form back." They rarely do.

Sometimes the men will say, "I have been feeling a little out of sorts. I lost my energy, it must be that I am getting older." Many times the man doesn't know he is depressed or will not admit it. He will rarely say to the doctor, "I feel depressed."

If they have a laundry list of symptoms with no diagnosed causes, some patients will refuse to accept the diagnosis of depression. Their symptoms are masqueraded as a substitute for depression and being anxious—still called psychosomatic symptoms. Many of these men will search out different doctors until they finally find one who gives them a spurious diagnosis that suits them, followed by B12 shots or herbs that make the patient feel better for a short while. Then they will say:

"At last I found a doctor who can help me, who made the right diagnosis." In the medical world this is called placebo treatment.

There is the story of a young woman who became depressed because her boyfriend, a medical school student, decided to break up with her. In those days the pharmaceutical companies gave out hundreds of drug samples to the med students. The samples included Maxidol and Ritalin. Both were used to keep the student awake for hours while studying for finals. The depressed girlfriend, who lived with the medical student, found a bottle of Maxidol—the ultimate upper—and swallowed ten of the pills thinking she was taking an overdosage of sleeping pills. She left a note: "I can't live without you."

Anyone else would have stayed awake for three days with those pills. She fell asleep and slept for 24 hours. This is a true example of the placebo effect. It is still used in hundreds of ways by charlatans and you can find them on the Internet promising to cure and take care of every symptom from which we suffer.

If the depression is due to a bad marriage it eventually leaves, once the marriage problems are resolved. Depressions resulting from the loss of a loved one, if not treated, can go on for years, resulting in sleep disturbances and a poor quality of life.

The sleep pattern of a depressed man is almost diagnostic. He goes to bed at 11:00 P.M. and awakens at 1:00 A.M., goes back to sleep and again is up at 4:00 A.M., and finally falls asleep at 6:00 A.M.—and for the rest of the morning the male feels exhausted. There are variations to this pattern but it is a helpful diagnostic clue for the spouse to diagnose depression. Once medications are used the doctor can use the sleep pattern to help guide him on gauging the efficacy of the treatment.

The cost of depression in the United States has been estimated at $43 billion per year, as a consequence of impaired job performance, medical, psychiatric, and pharmaceutical expenses.

More than 70 percent of patients who committed suicide visited a physician within two months of their death. These figures suggest that doctors were not aware that their patients were depressed and were thus at risk for suicide. And in the primary care setting, 25 percent of patients are depressed.

The spouse should question the cause if her man becomes impotent, which can be a symptom of depression. Cure the depression and the impotence may also be cured.

Alas, the appearance of depression might signal the presence of a cancer lurking somewhere in the body. Cancer of the pancreas may present itself with depression as the initial sign.

Substance abuse—above all, alcohol abuse—is another major cause of depression. Add to that a long laundry list of medical illness from infections (such as Lyme disease to an underactive thyroid). Any chronic illness can be accompanied with severe depression. Once the depression is treated the chronic or prolonged illness becomes easier to manage.

One-third of patients with non-psychiatric medical conditions suffer from some degree of depression when seen in a doctor's office.

Some men may complain of back problems for years, and are under the care of orthopedic surgeons, chiropractors, and generalists. X-ray studies and MRIs often will reveal signs of arthritis and bulging discs (which most of us have after a certain age), and the man will be treated for years with anti-inflammatory drugs, muscle relaxants, and manipulations for temporary relief, when, in reality, these men may be suffering from depression.

Headaches, neck pains, stomach problems, feeling flushed, chronic fatigue, chest pains, and so many other symptoms can be disguised symptoms of overt depression and anxieties.

Dr. David C. Steffens, an assistant professor psychiatry at Duke University, reported a link between strokes and depression. By studying the brain with MRIs in 3,600 subjects he and his colleagues discovered that the presence of depression after the age of 50 may indicate a silent stroke. This study was recently reported in the journal *Stroke*.

In my own practice, in dozens of male patients, depression was the most common finding right before a heart attack occurred. Without the obvious signs of cardiac disease mentioned above, major depression has shown a fourfold-increased risk of dying from heart disease.

Dr. Brenda Penninx reported at the Annual Meeting of the Gerontological Society in February, 2000, that older depressed patients between 55 and 85 had an excessive number of deaths from heart disease.

The spouse can be the first one to detect signs of her mate's hidden depression. We men can be such liars and actors that we can fool doctors but not our spouses. Men will not acknowledge they are depressed. Confront them and they will say, "You're crazy! I'm not depressed. I'm just tired of all that crap I have to put up with from everyone, including my wife. She drives me up the wall," et cetera.

The spouse who notices that her husband is moody, is suffering from a sleep disturbance, and, most critically, has lost his joy for most things, should be concerned. She should suggest or, if necessary, insist to her mate that he see his doctor for a physical, "just to see if everything is okay." She can call the doctor and tell him: "He will never admit to you, but he is depressed. Please don't tell him I called."

Now, that doctor, with this new information, and with the patient sitting in front of him, is empowered to practice the art of medicine. We must be careful not to use the wrong words or pose the wrong questions, because all can be lost as the patient soon will lose confidence in his doctor if he learns that the doctor and his wife have been chatting about him without his knowledge.

In most cases, it is very difficult to diagnose depression in a ten-or fifteen-minute office visit, and this is where the spouse can lay down the groundwork for the doctor.

After bypass operations, depression is a very common illness too often overlooked by the doctor, because the major symptom may be fatigue.

"After all, what do you expect after such a big operation? You're going to be washed out, perhaps for a year, with trouble concentrating and a loss of sexual appetite." These are the very words I once overheard from a doctor telling a patient two months after his open-heart surgery. Post-operative depression, not recognized by the doctor, can retard the patient's recovery. His life, instead of improving from having the surgery, may actually become worse. The depression can cause him to be fearful of doing anything. Some patients become confined to their home because they fear the chest will rip open and they also complain of the same pain as before the operation.

Now the cardiologist must perform a careful examination, as there is always the possibility that the grafts placed to bypass the obstruction are blocked and the patient also happens to be depressed.

Recently I saw a patient who had a successful operation but was afraid to walk and complained of being short of breath. All the heart tests were normal. However, once I started him on antidepressant medications he improved dramatically in a two-week period. He is now back at work.

Depression can occur after any surgery, even minor surgery like a tooth extraction. For women, hysterectomy can cause unrecognized depression for decades, sometimes masquerading as back pain, for example. For men, depression can follow knee surgery, back operations, or prostate surgery.

A solid antidepressant program, as outlined in the following, can make recovery faster and improve dramatically the quality of life.

There are commonly used medications that can cause depression, such as beta-blockers, thiazines, cimetidine, steroids, and anti-inflammatory agents, to mention a few.

Most depressions consist of three phases:

1. The acute phase, which lasts six-to-twelve weeks when treatment is started with antidepressants, will have a 75 percent cure. If not, a medication adjustment needs to be made and, certainly, an expert psychiatrist should be consulted. Many patients may respond without drugs. A high

percentage of prescriptions are not filled or the medications are not taken: "I'm not crazy, I don't need medication," is the common response of the male.

2. This is a continuation of phase 1. It should be continued for one year, with drug therapy lasting from four to nine months.

3. This is the chronic phase and usually requires medications for a very long period, sometimes indefinitely.

The spouse can help to see that her man takes his medication on a daily basis. Put it on the breakfast table. Also, take note of the fact that it is never a good idea to suddenly stop the medication without the doctor's approval and instructions.

Today, the first line of treatment used by the primary care doctor are Selective Seratonin Reupatake Inhibitors (SSRI), such as fluxoxetine, sertaline, citalopram, paroxetine, etc.

St. Johns wort has become a popular herb used in Europe extensively, and now in the United States. Recent studies have shown it is superior to a placebo, but much less effective than conventional antidepressant medications.

There are side effects that the spouse should be aware of such as restlessness, gastrointestinal symptoms, rash, and sensitivity to sunlight.

Before taking medications such as amiodarone, the statins, or verapamil, patients with heart disease—especially coronary artery disease—should know that they can be at risk of exacerbating their angina or arrhythmia. St. Johns wort acts as an inducer of the hepatic enzyme, cytochrome P450, and may cause these drugs to become less active.

Depression is an illness and needs to be approached as a medical and psychiatric illness. In many cases, counseling and psychotherapy alone may not be sufficient. I have known patients who have seen a therapist for years and remain depressed, while a program of antidepressants can make a dramatic, positive change in their lives.

The spouse can be a guiding light if her husband is depressed. She can encourage him to see a therapist and, if therapy alone is not helping, she should inquire if medication might better serve to lessen her husband's depression. A doctor who has experience with antidepressants, again, should only prescribe such medicine.

When I first started practicing in New Haven I was a medical consultant to a brilliant psychiatrist by the name of Henry Jarecki. Antidepressant pills, called tricycles, surfaced with the expert guidance of Dr. Detre, a renowned Yale psychiatrist; these doctors started to use them on a grand scale. It was similar to the miracle of penicillin curing the dreaded streptococcal infections, when the antidepressant tricyclic drugs attacked the chemical imbalance that causes depression. I witnessed hundreds of patients in the Doctor Jarecki and Dr. Detre Clinic in New Haven, who had been depressed and emotionally disabled for years, become viable again.

Unfortunately, in some cases, the depression is so severe that suicide is a constant threat, in spite of the medications, hospitalization, and electric convulsive therapy. The movie *One Flew over the Cuckoo's Nest* is a stark example of attempts to manage depression.

In some cases, suicide is perpetually on the mind of the patient and even expert psychiatrists can be fooled. A glaring example is Ernest Hemingway who was hospitalized for severe depression. The doctors decided he was ready to be discharged as his depression lifted. His wife, Mary, begged the doctors not to discharge him. She told the psychiatrists that Mr. Hemingway was fooling them. They would not listen and reassured Mary Hemingway. "Don't worry, he will be fine; you are just too anxious," they told her.

As soon as Ernest Hemingway returned home, that same day, he walked straight up to his hunting trophy room, took one of his shotguns off the wall, and blew his head off. There are many more examples of the same story.

Depression is a potentially lethal disease. Many times it is difficult to determine the severity of the depression. Unlike what we have available for other medical conditions, there are no tests that can gauge the seriousness of depression.

Chapter Twelve

The Formula for Increasing Your Man's Vitality

EVERY MAN I KNOW, regardless of age, would want a magic potion to increase his physical and mental strength, particularly his sexual vitality.

"Hey, doc, got something for me to give me more energy, some shot or something?"

"Right after dinner he sits on the couch, watches television and falls asleep—and he isn't old, 50 isn't old is it, doc?" So laments the concerned woman.

Barring any illness that is taking the spice out of the male, there are many things you can do to move your lover off the couch and, perhaps, into the bedroom if you so wish.

One of the major causes of loss of male vitality is smoking. Cigarettes kill more Americans each year than the total number of Americans killed in World War II, Korea, and the Vietnam War combined. It is a major cause for the male to become impotent, to develop heart disease, cancer, strokes, cancer of the throat and bladder, and to suffer from chronic fatigue, even loss of ambition.

Smoking also causes a disgusting odor to the skin and clothing, which recycles back into the body. It causes the same terrible effects on your spouse. Nicotine is a poison to the body. It travels to the brain, lungs, heart, kidney, and penis.

Cigarettes contain 10 mg of nicotine, and other poisons such as carbon monoxide, amine, and ammonia. Several puffs of a cigarette cause the heart to beat faster, constricts blood vessels, and makes the blood clot faster. It causes peripheral vascular disease, which results in pain in the legs when walking and exercise becomes difficult.

If you want your man to have more vigor, first and foremost he has to stop smoking cigarettes, cigars, or pipes. If you smoke, you too must give it up because he will suffer from the effects of second-hand smoke.

There are dozens upon dozens of gimmicks to induce the man to stop smoking—from hypnotism, to having his ear pierced with a copper filament, to smoking clinics, and "the patch."

It is not an easy task to convince a guy to give up smoking. If all fails, as it does so many times, try medications such as nicotine gum or the patch. It contains up to 4 mg of nicotine. It reduces the craving somewhat, and works by slowly withdrawing nicotine from the body. The best way to stop smoking is just to stop "cold turkey" and judiciously begin an exercise program with the guidance of your doctor.

Your spouse should use mouthwash four times a day to eradicate that chronic taste of smoke and continue to use a strong mouthwash for that phantom taste that lingers on after he gives up smoking. Otherwise the urge may not be so easy to suppress. Have all his clothing dry-cleaned; sanitize the room he smoked in with a thorough, strong cleaner. All these suggestions really work.

Finally, you could appeal to the male's fiduciary sense: *"If you give up smoking today I will give you $100,000 in ten to* *twenty years! If you take the five dollars a day you could spend on cigarettes and save it, you will have saved a great deal of money in twenty years. But you must place your cigarette money into a large saving can each day. At the end of the week you must take the money to a bank. At the end of each month you should buy one share of a blue chip stock."*

That is what convinced some of my poorer patients to do just that. Quality will prolong your life by ten years or more, as well as saving on doctor's bills and hospital bills. The best way to fight the HMOs and the pharmaceutical companies, and their outrageous fees, is to not smoke. If everyone would stop smoking the entire health care system would fall apart and become bankrupt—but you will be healthier and richer!

There are other measures a man can use to increase his zing. Reduce alcohol intake to a glass of wine or two ounces of hard alcohol per day. Not only will he sleep better and be more alert in the morning, but his sex life will blossom like a rich garden in the spring.

We humans have a marvelous internal pharmacy in our bodies. Dozens upon dozens of chemicals, hormones, and enzymes wait in anticipation to be called upon, to act in our benefit. They are our guardians of maintaining our well-being—unless they get destroyed or never used. Our brain cells that are concerned with memory, creativity, and intelligence are often not stimulated. It is a sad state for our society when so many brains are allowed to atrophy.

Luckily, we had brains like Albert Einstein and our Nobel Prize winners, whose brains were always stimulated to create. If our brains are not stimulated intellectually, they will not release those precious chemicals ready to serve us—and lessen fatigue as boredom is reduced—and thrust us to an active galloping life.

So you want more vitality in your spouse's life? Then start getting busy tapping into his internal pharmacy.

Exercise is the cheapest and most readily available positive stimulus for your spouse that will increase the vigor he yearns for. You have heard so much about the benefits of exercise, that you may feel "over-sold"—but it is all true and yet few Americans heed the free advice. For the Europeans it is part of their quotidian regimen.

Exercise increases the flow of blood in the body and turns on the adrenaline pump, the heart pump, the renal pump, and all the chemicals and transmitters of the brain including endorphins and helpful chemicals such as acetylcholine, which are necessary for brain memory transmission.

You don't have to start jogging miles at a time, or swimming the Long Island Sound, or wear out the treadmill, in order to achieve wonderful results. You will sleep better, stimulate oxidation of your fats, make more useful strong muscles for your body, increase the oxygen level in your blood (low levels of oxygen in your blood cause fatigue and loss of vigor), and use up excess sugar in the blood.

There are numerous formulae for an exercise prescription. The one I like the best is the exercise prescription of Dr. William B. Kannel who headed a twenty-five-year investigation in Framingham as follows:

1. It should be at least three times a week, or better yet, four or five times a week.
2. The exercise should be approximately of 20 minutes duration and it should be continuous. Numerous guidelines are recommended as to the intensity of the exercise: 60 to

80 percent of the maximum heart rate—subtract the patient's age from 220 and take 60, 70, or 80 percent of the figure as the heart rate at which the patient should exercise.

But from my point of view, you really don't need such strict guidelines unless your spouse is an obsessive-compulsive type who likes written guidelines. Exercise prescriptions usually fail after awhile. The treadmill, the exercycles and other mechanical aides gather dust and are expensive.

Do what you enjoy best. When you have finished your twenty-minute workout you should feel better, not worse. Exercising should be fun and not a medieval torture chamber. Tennis, reading, writing, and practicing medicine are my lifelines to an active, alert life.

Whenever possible it is nice to have your spouse join you for a brisk 40-minute walk three times or more per week. If you have an expert tennis player for a spouse, then it really becomes a more challenging and lasting exercise program.

Dancing is a wonderful romantic way to increase your spouse's vitality and all that follows. In the morning, before showering, it's fun to dance together to fast music for twenty minutes or so. It beats jogging. The day will begin with a smile before joining the hectic pace of the "dot com" world.

Sleep is the anodyne of the tensed-up, weary male—the way to make your body rest and get all the internal chemistry ready for action in the morning. Without it, there is not a chance to increase the vitality of your partner. Reread the section on insomnia in the earlier part of this book.

Sex is another way to stimulate those activator chemicals in the brain and body. Show me the couple with an active sex life and I will show you a very vigorous lifestyle. Viagra, or other injectable penile miracle drugs, can give a real boost to a flagging sex life.

How about vitamins and all those hundreds of herbs and potions that claim to increase your vitality "or your money back"? If it works, do it. But I can hardly recommend them without reservations.

Let's look back a few centuries to some of the cures recommended for rejuvenation of the tired soul. Centuries ago, the hucksters, who sold every concoction imaginable for the treatment of every medical condition, depended on the placebo effect. Placebo comes from the Latin "I shall please," and that is what it does.

About 35 percent or more of all placebo treatments are successful. Stories are legion about the power of positive thinking helping the body. Ulcer patients given saline injections into the arm, felt their pain disappear if the doctor told them, "This injection will cure your ulcer."

In the 1930s, the "Vitalizer" was a product sold in the United States until its producer was jailed for mail fraud. Soft drinks laced with cocaine, now illegal, were once sold in the United States.

Serge Voronoff, a wealthy Russian vodka manufacturer, started a luxurious villa clinic on the Italian Riviera. He made entire testicles available to rejuvenate men. Donors from young men were preferable, but chimpanzees were just as good. This bogus treatment cost the lives of thousands of chimps and made Voronoff a very rich man—but did little to rejuvenate the male. This practice still exists in places such as

South Korea, where bull testicles are mashed into a paste-like "delicacy" served to men to lower or increase their vigor.

We do use male hormone injections for men whose testosterone levels and sperm counts are low in order to restore their normal functions.

By now surely you have heard of Human Growth Hormone (HGH) injections for vigor and antiaging.

One of my friends injects himself twice daily. He is convinced that his lean body mass and skin thickness have improved, that his mind is sharper, and his sexual abilities have increased. He is 82 years old, and, frankly, this man had just as much energy before his injections. His mind was, and still is, as sharp as a tack and he plays a mean game of tennis. The injection causes fluid retention that, therefore, increases muscle diameter.

A Las Vegas–based company called Cenegenics, an antiaging center, as well as the American Academy of Antiaging Medicine based in Chicago, supply this Human Growth Hormone. There are thousands of hits on Internet sites offering HGH information and mail order sales.

This hormone is produced in our body by the pituitary gland, but the amount produced declines as we age. The Food and Drug Administration approved it for treating cases of pituitary failure, but not as an antiaging medication.

There are significant risks that come with this form of treatment, including heart failure, hypertension, and joint pain. It may also stimulate tumor formation and, as reported in an article in the *New England Journal of Medicine*, high doses of the hormone given to very sick patients increased their mortality rate. Likewise, the long-term effects are not yet known.

A prescription of HGH, depending on the dosage, can cost $9,000 to $17,000 per year.

I do not recommend this new treatment to restore vigor and prevent aging because there is little proof that it works. Assuredly we will hear more of this new "miracle" drug as more studies are performed.

The miracle of a vigorous life lies in ourselves and not in a pill.

Appendix

The Kra Diet

Being overweight—as 30 percent of Americans are—forces the heart to work harder in order to pump blood through all that extra fatty tissue. Excess body fat also can contribute to hardening of the arteries, high blood pressure, and other problems. For some heart patients, losing weight can literally be a matter of life or death. With the average American diet deriving 50 percent of its calories from fat, it's no wonder that heart disease continues to be the leading killer in the United States.

The health perils, not to mention the cosmetic challenge, of being too fat are not lost on most Americans. Each year, we spend an estimated $2 billion on weight-loss diets. In 90 percent of cases where the dieter does lose weight, however, the lost pounds are regained in relatively short order.

Having treated thousands of overweight heart patients over the last two decades, I have heard countless complaints about how difficult it is to stick to a low-caloric, low-fat diet. To help my patients, I developed a diet plan that is easy to follow and extremely effective. The plan basically entails alternating between a fish day and a vegetable day Monday through Saturday, and rewarding yourself with a poultry or meat meal on Sunday. The Kra Diet includes ample helpings of pasta, breads, fruits, and grains, and certain oils, nuts, and other foods that have been scientifically shown to lower blood cholesterol. The diet also encourages a liberal use of spices to prevent your meals from being too bland.

If you are currently free of heart disease, following the Kra Diet will reduce your risk of developing heart problems in the future. If your coronary arteries are already narrowed, following my diet could reverse the disease process by reducing the amount of cholesterol plaque clogging your coronary arteries.

My diet achieves this goal by reducing your fat intake to approximately 10 percent, or less, of consumed calories. You will also lower your daily cholesterol intake from the average 800 mg to less than 200 mg. By reducing dietary fat, the Kra Diet aims to lower your overall blood cholesterol level by 30 percent, your LDL level by at least 20 percent and your triglyceride level by 30 to 40 percent. As explained in Chapter 3, LDL and triglycerides contribute to atherosclerosis.

WHY DIETS FAIL

Before reading the particulars of the Kra Diet, it helps to understand why diets fail. A major reason is that dieters often underestimate the number of calories they take in each day, according to a recent study in the *New England Journal of Medicine*. Counting calories is a mainstay of most diet programs, including mine. It therefore is crucial to keep an accurate daily log of how many calories you ingest in order to avoid this trap.

Another trap people fall into is conjuring up excuses for gaining weight. My patients often attribute their weight gain to holidays, weddings, birthdays, cocktail parties, or business luncheons. Other patients cite unhappiness in their lives as a reason for gaining weight. For them, the only activity that seems to bring any pleasure is eating. Overeaters Anonymous, Weight Watchers, and other support groups have helped many people develop better eating habits.

Some patients complain that they hardly eat anything but cannot lose even a pound. Eating too little fools your body into thinking it is starving; the body's response to caloric withdrawal is to slow down the metabolism. This means you are not burning as many calories as you normally would as you go about your normal activities.

Another reason people don't lose weight is because they fail to couple their diet with exercise. Even if you make no changes in your caloric intake, increasing your level of physical activity will enable you to burn more body fat than you are gaining.

HOW MANY CALORIES DO I NEED?

To calculate your daily caloric requirement, multiply your ideal weight by 10. For example, a woman who should weigh 130 pounds needs at least 1,300 calories a day. In order to lose one pound, you must burn 3,500 to 4,000 calories. If you use up 1,500 calories a day with normal activity, and another 500 or so with exercise, while taking in only 1,500 calories, you will have a net loss of 500 calories a day. At the end of seven days, you will have lost 1 pound. In a month, you will have lost up 4 to 4.5 pounds. In one year, you theoretically could lose 52 pounds on the Kra Diet, although most people will shed a lesser but respectable 25 to 30 pounds.

KNOWING THE NUMBERS

As you embark on the Kra Diet, these basic facts should help you better track your caloric intake:

** One gram of fat contains 9 calories. To find out how many calories of fat in the food you are about to eat, look at the label and multiply the number of grams of fat by nine.
** One gram of sugar contains 4 calories.

GETTING STARTED

Before you begin the diet, stock up on herbs and spices, such as basil, curry, chili powder, bay leaves, caraway seeds, cloves, ginger, garlic, mustard, nutmeg, oregano, peppercorns, sage, thyme, saffron, and any other spices you like. Spices greatly enhance the flavor of foods while adding no fat and very few calories to your meals.

Also buy some walnuts, a good source of Omega-3 fatty acid, the same that's in fish oil. Some of my physician friends munch on walnuts every day in order to lower their blood cholesterol and reduce their risk of heart attack.

WHAT TO EAT

Other items to buy for the Kra Diet are brown rice, black beans, low-fat yogurt, chickpeas, kidney beans, lentils, lima beans, great northern beans, and pinto beans. Also buy high-fiber foods, including oats, potatoes, barley, rice bran, wheat bran, graham crackers, and whole-grain breads such as rye and pumpernickel. Don't forget the fresh fruits and vegetables: apples, plums, peas, carrots, cabbage, broccoli, oranges, tangerines, and tomatoes, to name a few. Grains, fruit, and vegetables should be eaten every day. (Vegetable haters may enjoy low-salt vegetable juices, which are packed with nutrients.)

Pasta, another nutritious low-fat food, also can be eaten daily. Eating pasta with garlic sautéed in olive oil is particularly good for your heart. The Italians eat plenty of it, and they boast the lowest heart-attack rate in Europe. Olive oil is high in monounsaturated fat, which lowers blood cholesterol. Garlic also is getting a very good reputation for lowering the incidence of coronary artery disease. Studies expected to prove garlic's health benefits are under way in Germany.

Foods to eliminate from your diet include egg yolks and butter. Use cooking oils sparingly, except for olive oil which should be included in as many meals as possible. Avoid coconut, palm, and other tropical oils because they are very high in saturated fats, which raise the blood cholesterol level. Food labels will tell you whether tropical oils are present.

Ideally, a vegetarian diet is best for the heart. But I have included in the Kra Diet fish, poultry, and small quantities of red meat to make it appealing to a wider audience. Most people find it difficult to maintain a strict vegetarian diet because they read it diminishes their quality of life.

My simple "modified vegetarian" diet is designed to be followed six days a week. On the seventh day, you may reward yourself with your favorite meal. You may have a glass of wine each day with dinner or lunch. As mentioned earlier, the Kra Diet alternates a total vegetarian day with a fish day. Chicken or beef days are sprinkled in once a week. Vegetables should be eaten every day, including the fish day and on the seventh "reward" day. Meat is permitted only once a week. Poultry cannot be used on the fish or vegetarian days. Three ounces of chicken without the skin has as much cholesterol (60 mg) as three ounces of beef. A serving should be no bigger than the palm of your hand.

The fish day need not be boring. Seafood is actually quite delicious if it's fresh and prepared properly. You may use shellfish anytime you like, but eat seafood either baked or broiled, not fried. Some people dislike seafood because of the smell and taste. Using lots of spices or baking fish in parchment paper masks the fishy taste. For example, you can brush scrod with olive, canola, or peanut oil, add some wine, garlic, and chives, and bake it in parchment paper or just broil it in the oven. You can use a small amount of a brown sauce to give your fish a little zest.

On vegetarian days, variety is key. You can stir-fry vegetables in a wok with spices and olive oil. You can steam vegetables and serve them over rice. You can add vegetables and legumes to soup, which is a nutritious addition to any meal. For example, lentil soup cooked with onions, tomatoes, carrots, and thyme is delicious. If you don't have time to cook soup from scratch, there is a growing variety of low-salt canned soups available. On vegetarian days, you can whip up some pasta with tomato sauce or olive oil and garlic in minutes. Or use cholesterol-free eggs to make a vegetable omelet cooked in olive or safflower oil.

Breakfast is a natural with the Kra Diet. It can include whole grain cold cereals with skim milk, hot oatmeal, fruit juice, and toasted whole-grain bread with jam.

GET ENOUGH FLUIDS

Be sure to drink two to three glasses of water in the morning and again in the afternoon. Keeping your fluid intake adequate promotes good kidney function and decreases your desire for food. Water retention can be negligible if you maintain a low-salt diet.

Try not to skip meals, especially breakfast, because it gives you energy and makes you less hungry for lunch. Please consult your doctor before starting this diet

---

SAMPLE MENUS:

FISH DAY

Breakfast: Bran flakes; orange juice or a fruit; one slice of whole-wheat, pumpernickel, or rye bread with low-fat cottage cheese, farmer cheese, low-fat American cheese, or goat cheese; a slice of tomato; coffee. Eating a low-fat bran muffin with jelly in lieu of the bread will further curb your lunchtime appetite.

Lunch: Tuna (water-packed) with onions, garlic, and tomatoes on a green salad; two water crackers. Tuna can be substituted with canned salmon, sardines, smoked trout, shrimp, scallops, oysters, or lobster salad with reduced-fat mayonnaise; low-fat yogurt for dessert.

Dinner: Any fish with spices, baked or broiled, served with brown rice and lima beans, or with dill sauce (made with grated onions, chopped dill, black pepper, lemon juice, and yogurt); salad of tomatoes with olive oil and vinegar, chives, garlic, and Dijon mustard; frozen low-fat yogurt, low-fat ice cream, or Italian ices for dessert; coffee or tea.

VEGETABLE DAY

Breakfast: Juice, bran flakes, banana, sliced dark bread with jelly, farmer or low-fat cottage cheese; coffee with low-fat milk.

Lunch: Large glass of salt-free vegetable juice; salad with olive oil, lentils, chives, and tomatoes; vegetable soup; crackers with tahini or hummus; unsalted air-popped popcorn.

Dinner: Lentil or minestrone soup; stir-fried vegetables of your choice or steamed vegetables with olive oil, garlic, pepper, and chives; brown rice or potatoes (not fried), or pasta with tomato sauce; two slices of dark bread; glass of wine; sherbet, Jell-O, or fruit for dessert.

SEVENTH DAY

On the seventh day, you may eat a lean steak, chicken, or veal, some cheese, or most anything else you crave. Be sure to include grains, such as bread and complex carbohydrates, such as beans. Half an egg is permissible, but avoid butter and whole milk, and don't let your daily caloric count exceed 1,500.

At end of six weeks, the Kra Diet should reduce your overall blood cholesterol level to below 190, and your LDL to 130. If this has not happened, I recommend cholesterol-lowering medications if you have coronary artery disease or peripheral vascular disease.

This diet requires some imagination and creativity on your part. I have given you the outline; you must write the script.

And, as with all diet programs, consult your doctor before embarking on it. People who have tried this diet enjoy the relative freedom it offers. Over the past ten years, I am pleased to report that it has worked wonders for many of my patients. I am hopeful it will do the same for you.

Index